Thinking Outside the Voice Box

Thinking Outside the Voice Box

Adolescent Voice Change in Music Education

Bridget Sweet

OXFORD
UNIVERSITY PRESS

OXFORD
UNIVERSITY PRESS

Oxford University Press is a department of the University of Oxford. It furthers the University's objective of excellence in research, scholarship, and education by publishing worldwide. Oxford is a registered trade mark of Oxford University Press in the UK and certain other countries.

Published in the United States of America by Oxford University Press
198 Madison Avenue, New York, NY 10016, United States of America.

CIP data is on file at the Library of Congress
ISBN 978–0–19–091638–1 (pbk.)
ISBN 978–0–19–091637–4 (hbk.)

Hardback printed by Bridgeport National Bindery, Inc., United States of America

This book is dedicated to all adolescents.

May you always feel inspired and empowered to sing with your true voice.

May you always feel empowered and worthy to speak with your inner voice.

And to my beautiful family. I love you all so much.

CONTENTS

ACKNOWLEDGMENTS

With Gratefulness

Norm Hirschy: I think your name is in more Acknowledgments sections of music books than anyone else's, and there is a reason: you are *amazing.* Thank you for all of your encouragement to pursue this project, for your ability to not only see my vision but help me make it better, and for your fabulous and complex sense of humor. You "get me" and constantly empower me to stick with my own perspective. Thanks, Norm. I am endlessly appreciative for all you do and look forward to more projects together.

Thank you to Jane Zanichkowsky for your keen eye and hours of careful, meticulous work. I am so appreciative of Lauralee Yeary, Leslie Johnson, Rajesh Kathamuthu, and all of the editorial and production staff who assisted with the production stages of my book. You have all helped to make this book stronger and I am very grateful.

Thank you to Dr. Elizabeth Cassidy Parker for your collaboration, insight, graciousness, patience, humor, and brilliance, but most important, your friendship. Working with you on all of our varied projects has been a highlight of my career and I look forward to all yet to come.

Thank you to Dr. Louis Bergonzi for your imagination and creative way of thinking about teaching music and honoring adolescents. I really enjoyed the experience of our joint project and am proud of the work we were able to do.

Thank you to my amazing artist sister, Kate Cosgrove, for her original illustrations of the larynx and vocal fold layers featured in chapter 2. Your work is (as usual) stunning, and I am *so proud* to include it here. You are my dearest friend and I love you very much.

Yvonne Redman, not only are you an incredible musician, you are one of the most inquisitive, thoughtful, and caring people I know. I love geeking out with you about the voice and look forward to many more conversations . . . especially while we get our nails done.

Thank you to Adam Kruse for providing me with your photography skills and for your work within hip-hop that spurred my initial thinking about chapter 4. I am appreciative of Michael Silver who taught me about Paulo Abel do Nascimento, which led me to new considerations of the voice. I am also grateful for the speech and hearing specialists who kindly helped me during my construction of chapter 1: Pasquale Bottalico, Tina Childress, Mary Flaherty, Lori J. Leibold, and Brian Monson.

There are many people who have influenced or supported me in countless positive ways, and for them I am *hugely* thankful: Janet Barrett, Christine Benway, Deb Borton, Amy Davis, Tami Draves, Sean Grier, Colleen Hartung, Lisa Koops, Barry Long, Jeremy Manternach, Deb McMartin-Finkel, Jeananne Nichols, Anne Nispel, Sarah Reynertson, Vicki Sandstrom, Mary Ann Schmedlen, and Sheri Tulloch. Thank you for everything, my dear and wonderful friends.

I am a lucky gal to have such a wonderful and supportive family. Special thanks to my momola, Marsha Cosgrove; my dad, Patrick Cosgrove, and his wife, Patricia; Deb, Tony, Chris, Juniper, Tiny, Erin, Sophia, Ava, Vivian, and Abbey.

My two fabulous children, Luke and Evelyn, you are *the* greatest people I know and you constantly help me to be my best, silly self. You are both *so funny* and you bring such joy and sparkle and perspective to my days. You truly make this world a much brighter, better place. I love you forever and now let's go cuddle more.

My husband, Jason, knows *all* that went into this book more than anyone else in the world. Your kindness and support, patience and love have allowed this project to come to fruition; I'm not sure how it could have happened without you. There is little that I can do to adequately express my appreciation for all, but I put a *Deadpool* quote in a choral music education book, so that's a start. I love you, my zing.

Introduction

Framing

This is not a book of vocal exercises for changing voices or a book of repertoire suggestions. This book is different from most other books about voice change because the intention is to encourage new and less orthodox ways of thinking about the adolescent changing voice. A goal is to provide choral music teachers (or anyone interested in the changing voice) the opportunity to step away from typical considerations of vocal change and reflect on the bigger picture of the experience for adolescents. *Then*, armed with this wider scope and comprehension of the true complexity of adolescent voice change, choral music educators can more judiciously comb through the many resources for vocal exercises and repertoire. So again, this is not a book of techniques, as it will go much bigger and much deeper than that. And as Charles Dickens wrote at the very start of *A Christmas Carol*, "This must be distinctly understood, or nothing wonderful can come of the story I am going to relate" (1843).

Adolescent voice change was not a topic of lengthy discussion during my undergraduate music education program, so I entered the profession with K-12 choral-general teaching licensure but with limited understanding and knowledge of the changing voice. My first teaching position involved seventh- to ninth-grade choirs in a junior high school, and my students' voices were all over the voice change map. My second year as a choral teacher began in a different school district from the first, where I taught sixth- to eighth- grade choirs; again, issues of voice change remained front and center. I think back to those early classes of mine and I feel a twinge of guilt for my former students. I know that I did not un-educate anyone or teach in ways that would lead to vocal damage or dangerous singing habits, but I *certainly* could have done more to inform and support my female and male students as they navigated voice change.

Over the following years I completed a summer master's program in music education and began digging into literature and published research pertaining to the changing voice. Each fall I returned to my own middle school classroom more prepared to work with singers undergoing voice change based on what I had read and studied during the previous summer's master's courses. I have continued to read about and research this topic—and vocal health and function in general—and greatly respect the process of voice change as a whole-body experience for adolescents, both female and male.

When I tell people that I really like working with adolescent singers, responses range from "I could never work with that age group" or "Too much going on with voice change for me" to a blatant "Blech." Such comments are really frustrating, especially because few of these people have truly learned about teaching adolescent singers, and their overall perceptions of adolescents are rooted in misunderstanding or no understanding at all. On the other hand, there are many teachers who enjoy working with adolescents and embrace the challenges of voice change in their work. I feel compelled to take a moment and acknowledge the work of music educators who genuinely enjoy working with this age group and guarantee three things about these people:

1. They are not crazy for loving working with singers whose voices are changing. There is nothing wrong with them. A person can simply really enjoy such students.
2. If they work with middle school singers, it does not mean that they are not good enough to secure a high school choral position.
3. Teachers can work as middle school music educators for their entire lives and be happy and fulfilled. They do not have to leave a middle school position for a high school position or something deemed more prestigious if they enjoy what they are doing.

I have two related stories from my own experiences.

First, after I received my undergraduate degree in music education, I attended the annual music education conference in my state and ran into many college friends and educators. I proudly told one person from my past that I was working as a choir teacher at a middle school and his immediate reply was, "Oh. You couldn't get a high school job?" I was infuriated because of all that was implied by his comment, mostly that middle school was inferior and not worthy of my time.

Second, while teaching at the University of Illinois, I received a message from a former music education student who was doing an amazing job teaching middle school choir. The high school position in her district was opening and she wondered if she should apply. The conversation went like this:

M.S. TEACHER: The high school position is open. Should I apply?
ME: Do you want to apply?
M.S. TEACHER: No. But it is a high school position, so. . .
ME: Do you want to leave middle school and teach high school?
M.S. TEACHER: No. I *love* my job. I just didn't know if it would look bad if it came open and I didn't take it. I don't really want to leave my middle school.
ME: So don't leave your middle school.
[She decided to stay at the middle school and is very happy. End scene.]

The bottom line is that we all have our niche, and if adolescents are your niche, then so be it! Celebrate it! Shout it from the rooftops! Do *not* feel ashamed by it or inferior because of it. Adolescents need more overt and visible allies in this world, and who better to help on the front line than you?

I firmly believe that every age group has positive aspects and challenging aspects associated with it, whether we are considering pre-K children, high school students, or adult musicians. The adolescent age group is no different, and there are really lovely aspects of this population, as well as challenging characteristics. Voice change is just one small part of working with adolescents, but it is often the biggest reason why choral educators discount or shy away from the age group. I find that discouraging. Voice change should not scare music teachers away from working with middle-level singers; it should be understood and draw people closer to the age group. Is it always easy? Absolutely not! But rather than focusing strictly on struggle, angst, and challenge, why not focus on the great moments of success and perseverance, fascination and intrigue, hard work and levity? *That* is the view of voice change and adolescents (and adolescence) that I desire to reinforce in our profession of choral music education. Worthwhile is not the same as easy, but *wow,* can the process be one fantastic adventure for both choral teachers and students.

Singers with changing voices spring up in upper elementary school, are pretty much the norm in middle school, and are definitely part of early high school. Some singers may experience vocal development even after high school, although that has more to do with the instrument's solidifying and fortifying than with growing in size (more on that to come). There is no magic switch that is flipped as students enter or leave middle school or junior high school that suddenly initiates or resolves vocal challenges related to laryngeal development. To complicate matters, residual emotions and memories connected to voice change experiences—especially negative ones—can outlast physiological challenges with the voice and greatly influence future voice use. As such, voice change should be a topic of interest for choral music educators and voice teachers at multiple school levels. The stereotype that *only* middle school or junior high teachers have to work with such singers is just not true.

In this book I situate adolescent voice change among a number of other related factors, including physical development, biological growth, psychological consideration, societal expectation, identity formation, and music education. It is also important to consider findings from published research in choral music education, and much of that will be referenced as well. My purpose for writing this book is to encourage choral educators to foster and maintain a more holistic perspective of female and male voice change. And then from there, after reading this book, go forth and consider your own teaching practices and methods in new, multifaceted ways to better meet the varied needs of your own adolescent singers. I firmly believe that adolescent singers are best served if we do our best to understand *them* first and inlay the music second; students' needs are primary, and musical needs are secondary.

An important place to start is actually not with the voice, but by first considering a wider perspective on adolescence. In chapter 1, topics include scrutiny, general body growth and coordination, adolescent brain and cognitive development, hearing mechanism growth, and emotion in order to begin thinking holistically about adolescence, of which voice change is a part. Vocal anatomy and physiology are unpacked in detail in chapter 2, as are physical changes that occur in the larynx during adolescent voice change. Implications of hormone fluctuation and premenstrual vocal syndrome for female singers also are addressed. Chapter 3 focuses on ideas of resolve that are essential to the navigation of voice change; perseverance is explored under the designations of grit, vulnerability, and relentlessness. An additional section considers perseverance in practice and provides strategies for music students and educators to utilize during voice change challenges and beyond. Chapter 4 examines the ways popular knowledge, understanding, and misunderstanding of voice change are largely perpetuated by mainstream media. Portrayals of voice change distributed via music, television, movies, and games have contributed to a simulacrum of adolescent voice change, a situated reality not based in fact but accepted in pop culture. This idea is explored through examination and distillation of episodes of *The Brady Bunch*, *The Wonder Years*, and *The Goldbergs*, popular television shows that represented a span of more than forty years, each with an episode focused on the adolescent changing voice. Chapter 5 provides a larger scope of voice classification systems and other foundational ideas in choral music education through examination of some of the most eminent works in the profession by Emil Behnke and Lennox Brown, Duncan McKenzie, Irvin Cooper and Karl O. Kuersteiner, Richard Luchsinger and Godfrey E. Arnold, Frederick J. Swanson, John Cooksey, and Lynne Gackle. In this chapter I also challenge choral educators to consider voice classification systems more as guidelines for helping teachers assist adolescent singers through voice change than as steadfast stages through which all voices pass, so that the systems are utilized as supporting tools to help guide the process of voice change rather than label adolescent singers' changing voices. The goal of chapter 6 is to discuss emerging considerations of adolescent voice change beyond classification systems and provide new food for thought about working with the adolescent changing voice. Sections of chapter 6 address female singers, voice change from the perspective of professional musicians who identify as transgender, and ideas for working with changing voices beyond classification systems, especially with regard to approaching choral repertoire. The Additional Resources section at the conclusion of the book was compiled with the intention of identifying additional items that may further enhance or enrich explorations of topics discussed in this book.

DISCLAIMERS

Hormonal Discrepancies

Before getting too far into this book, I have a few disclaimers. I acknowledge that human hormonal climates vary greatly from person to person, and those climates affect the sex of one's voice. As stated in the voice science article "Sex Hormones and the Female Voice" in *Journal of Voice*:

> A person's sex depends on his or her genetic mapping, XX for woman or XY for man, but the sexual genotype does not necessarily correspond to the sex of the voice. *The hormonal climate determines the sex of the voice.* The absence of androgens at puberty leads to a feminine voice. The presence of the same hormones at any stage in life will give a masculine voice. (Abitbol, Abitbol, & Abitbol, 1999, p. 433, emphasis in original)

With the understanding that cases of atypical hormone levels exist, discussion about voice change throughout this book pertains to adolescents with "typical" hormone levels, especially in dealing with anatomy and physiology. I acknowledge that there may be exceptions to what is discussed in this book as a result of each person's unique hormonal composition.

Typical versus Atypical Chromosomal Composition

In addition to a shared consensus about hormone levels, it is important that we also agree on the definition of *sex chromosomes*:

> Sex chromosome: either of a pair of chromosomes that determine whether an individual is male or female. The sex chromosomes of human beings and other mammals are designated by scientists as X and Y. In humans the sex chromosomes comprise one pair of the total of 23 pairs of chromosomes. The other 22 pairs of chromosomes are called autosomes. Individuals having two X chromosomes (XX) are female; individuals having one X chromosome and one Y chromosome (XY) are male. This path to maleness or femaleness originates at the moment of meiosis, when a cell divides to produce gametes, or sex cells having half the normal number of chromosomes. During meiosis the male XY sex-chromosome pair separates and passes on an X or a Y to separate gametes; the result is that one-half of the gametes (sperm) that are formed contains the X chromosome and the other half contains the Y chromosome. The female has two X chromosomes, and all female egg cells normally carry a single X. The eggs fertilized by X-bearing sperm become females (XX), whereas those fertilized by Y-bearing sperm become males (XY). (https://www.britannica.com/science/sex-chromosome)

A percentage of the human population genetically identifies outside of the typical sex chromosomal composition of XX or XY. Turner syndrome is caused by the absence of all or part of the second X chromosome in some or all of the cells of the body; it only affects girls and women (http://www.turnersyndrome.org/). Klinefelter syndrome is a condition that affects men in which an extra X chromosome is present; a person with this syndrome is also known as an XXY male (http://www.klinefeltersyndrome.org/). Additional chromosomal disorders include Triple X syndrome (also called trisomy X), in which a female has three X chromosomes, and XYY syndrome (also known as Jacobs syndrome, XYY karyotype, or YY syndrome), in which a male has an extra copy of a Y chromosome in each of his cells. Although having a chromosomal condition does not guarantee that an adolescent will experience voice change differently than those with typical XX or XY chromosomal makeup, discussion in this book pertains to "typical" chromosomal composition. Therefore, there may be exceptions to what is discussed for some people, especially those diagnosed with atypical chromosomal structures.

Endocrinal Influence

Each of us has an endocrine system that contains all of the glands in our body that make our hormones. Across the centuries there have been documented cases of atypical endocrine function in males and females that has affected their glands and, thus, impacted vocal development:

> The hormonal glands with internal secretion play an important role in the development of voice types. Despite a wide range of variability, it is a fact that exceptionally low female voices are associated with a tendency to virilization. Conversely, *underdevelopment of the male gonads* contributes to the development of abnormally high male voices. (Luchsinger & Arnold, 1965, p. 102, emphasis in original)

Virilization is a condition in which females develop characteristics associated with male hormones, such as muscle bulk, deep voice, body hair, and so forth. It could also be referenced as masculinization.

Castrato. The castrato—a male classical singer with a voice equivalent to a soprano's—is one of the most prominent examples of the intersection of historical vocal practice and the endocrine system. The word *castrato* refers to the fact that these singers were castrated as young men, meaning that their testicles were removed before puberty so that hormones could not trigger voice change; thus, the male child's voice was preserved. The decline of this practice began following the 1870 ban on the use of castrato voices by Pope Leo XIII (r. 1878–1903). One of the last castrato singers was Alessandro Moreschi, who died at age 63 in 1922. He was the only castrato to have recorded his voice, and you can hear him sing after a quick online search. I find his voice to be both beautiful and haunting.

Conditional factors. Other factors such as malnourishment and environmental conditions can influence function of the endocrine system and impact adolescent vocal development. In his paper "Voice Change in Human

Biological Development" Herbert Moller examined vocal development and the influence of external factors, specifically during the Middle Ages:

> It appears that the maturation of the vocal apparatus was impeded in the same way as was growth in height due to nutritional, environmental, and possibly behavioral factors. During the Middle Ages the great majority of Europe's population remained shorter than their modern descendants, including even the reputedly tall Scandinavians. It has been claimed that "laryngeal growth is significantly correlated with growth in body height." Under medieval health conditions and consumption levels the voice mechanism—the vocal folds, muscles, cartilages, and bones that function in the throat and mouth area in the production of sounds—was less developed than it is today. (Moller, 1985, p. 247)

In his 1970 article "Age of Boys' Puberty in Leipzig, 1727–49, as Indicated by Voice Breaking in J. S. Bach's Choir Members," historical researcher S. F. Daw reported his suspicion that lack of nutrition and wartime conditions during a key time in adolescence greatly delayed the onset of voice change in young males in Leipzig at that time. He wrote,

> One explanation of this would appear to be the poverty caused in Saxony by the War of the Austrian Succession (1740–1748). Leipzig, the second largest town in the principality, suffered the imposition of crippling taxes, and in 1745 was occupied for about three weeks by a Prussian army, which forced the citizens to supply it with provisions. All of this must have affected the diet and possibly the health of the Thomasschule scholars. Deaths at the school increased markedly during those years. (Daw, 1970, pp. 88–89)

What Daw ultimately found was that during this period Bach's choirboys did not begin voice change until at least age 17 and sometimes age 18. This was a remarkable finding, especially when he compared this historical data with 1959 health statistics from London which reported that adolescent male voices were changing at the age of 13.3 years.

Endocrinological castrato. Another thread of this conversation is the endocrinological castrato. For such males, the endocrine system does not "kick in" and typical hormone production does not happen, preventing a boy's voice from changing to that of an adult male. Two well-known endocrinological castrati (now referred to as male sopranos) in today's music industry include Michael Maniaci (born in 1976) and Radu Marian (born in 1977). One of the most famous endocrinological castrati was singer Paulo Abel do Nascimento, who passed away in 1992 at age 35. He was the 15th child in his very poor Brazilian family and, as a result of an extreme lack of nutrition, his endocrine system never fully initiated puberty and his voice never changed.

Discussion of the endocrine system in relation to adolescent voice change is important because it challenges the idea that every person goes through a voice change. It also might suggest that voice change is a privileged development, associated with a certain kind of situational able-bodiedness. Similar to the above disclaimers regarding hormones and chromosomes, I acknowledge that as a result of endocrinological factors, not everyone will experience a "typical" voice change during adolescence. However, in this book I focus on adolescent female and male singers who are experiencing the symptoms and expectations of a "typical" adolescent voice change.

Transgender Voice Change

In chapter 6 I include perspectives on voice change from professional musicians who identify as transgender. There are also many, many concepts throughout the book that apply to our work with LGBTQ+ singers, especially those transitioning to a new gender or vocal identity. While I do not address transgender voice change at length in this book, I do believe that all people have a right to use their literal and figurative voices in our choirs and that, no matter what, *everyone* is important.

CHAPTER 1
The Adolescent

Recently I was invited to be the guest clinician for a school district's new young men's choral festival. The original composition of the festival changed over the course of planning and, long story short, I ended up with a group of 79 fourth- through ninth-grade male singers. It was a diverse group of boys and young men who were (mostly) excited for a Saturday full of singing. We discussed vocal anatomy and voice change; we danced to music; we used our voices in a myriad of ways. The singers were loud and wiggly, raw and polished, playful and serious, and as the day progressed, the endearing odor of sweaty adolescent filled the space and we concluded the day with a wonderful concert brimming with adolescent sincerity.

However, one moment during the day was so poignant and powerful that, in my mind, it defined the entire experience. In the front row of chairs stood a very tiny fourth grade boy, whom we will call "James." It was quite clear that James was overwhelmed by everything, especially the size of the other boys in attendance. He stood so still in the front row clutching his white three-ring binder of music with his Mickey Mouse winter coat zipped up to his chin long after rehearsal had begun, even after other teachers and I encouraged him to join in and make himself comfortable. At one point, James did remove his coat and was trying to follow his music, but was so lost. As I started to walk to him to provide some help, a seventh grade boy from the back row, "Alex," emerged from nowhere, crouched beside James and said, "Can I help you? You seem like you could use a little extra help." Alex stayed with James for a while and helped him get on track with his music before retreating to his place again in the back row. And every so often, Alex checked in with James to make sure he was okay.

I was so struck by the completely unsolicited help that Alex provided to James. Alex helped him because he *needed* help. It was simply the right thing to do. And it was executed in such a caring and sweet way that I couldn't help but be reminded of my own small son and my hope that others are as kind to him when he needs help. As the day continued, I saw many additional moments when the boys took care of each other, from sharing music to helping others match pitch to applauding and high-fiving one another for little and big efforts. During the concert that evening, I made a point to tell the audience that they have amazing students who demonstrated numerous acts of humanity towards one another. I may or may not have said, "And anyone who says that adolescent boys can't be compassionate . . . well . . . screw them" but it's a bit foggy. I do remember the look on the faces in the crowd—grins and smiles and nodding "yes" with their heads and applause. They know what their adolescent students are capable of and they are proud of their adolescents. It was important for them to know that someone recognized it in their child as well.

When working with adolescents of all genders, I often see positive gestures and action towards others. These moments continually reinforce my admiration for the age group, for I know and believe that adolescents are capable of carrying out amazing acts of kindness and humanity, they know right from wrong, and they have much to offer the world. I have seen it in action. Unfortunately, these sorts of positive interactions and gestures are overwhelmingly eclipsed by stories of angst, risk-taking, and bad decision-making in the media and on television, reinforcing the stereotype that adolescents are generally troubled, challenging, and brooding people. Based on their reaction to my comments, that crowd at the concert knew what the larger society generally thinks about their adolescent child and it is unpleasant. Ian McMahan wrote the following in his book *Adolescence*:

> I dropped by a large bookstore and browsed in the Parenting department. The books were arranged by age. On the first shelves, I noticed such titles as *The Magic Years*, *How to Raise a Happy Baby*, and *Kids Are Worth It*. The covers featured cute, smiling babies and attractive, smiling parents. Then I moved a few feet to the right, to the Adolescence section. Some of the titles caught my eye: *The Roller Coaster Years*, *How to Keep Your Teenager Out of Trouble*, *How to Stop the Battle with Your Teenager*, *How to Keep Your*

> *Teenager from Driving You Crazy, Yes, Your Teen Is Crazy!* Clearly, the idea that adolescence has to be a time of "storm and stress" is alive and well and living at Barnes & Noble! (McMahan 2008, 156)

I cannot count the number of times that I've received a negative reaction from someone when I tell them how much I enjoy working with adolescents—the instances are truly countless from over the years. So a large factor in my becoming a music teacher educator has been to change the minds of people about adolescents and adolescence. I am on a self-appointed mission to fight deficit perceptions of adolescents. To glaringly point out their senses of humor, wit, intelligence, innocence, wickedness, compassion and empathy to others so that they are viewed in different lights and more supported and celebrated. Adolescence is a remarkably wonderful and important time of transition, as the recent movie *Inside Out* shows us. And although adolescence is not easy, navigating from child to adult can be a very positive experience if we continue to keep the perception glass half-full. (Sweet, 2016b)

I wrote this book in order to promote new ways of thinking about adolescents and their experiences of voice change, beginning with the acknowledgment that voice change is a long and complex process. As mentioned in the introduction, voice change is not restricted to people aged eleven through thirteen. There is no magic switch that is flipped as students progress from middle school to high school that suddenly enables the voice in all ways, eliminates breathiness, and abruptly allows for pristine precision in singing. Voice change is a physiological process that lasts many years and involves the psyche and emotions, which tend to remain the most vivid aspects of voice change long after physiological growth is finished.

This book actually starts not with the voice but by first considering the larger picture of adolescent development and noting our reactions to the varied facets of adolescence. As Nancy Lesko writes in *Act Your Age! A Cultural Construction of Adolescence*, "If we want to see adolescence differently, we must first understand the ways we currently see, feel, think, and act toward youth, or we will merely tinker with the reigning practices" (2012, p. 8). Awareness of the bigger picture of adolescence allows us to more meaningfully meet the needs of singers undergoing voice change. I like using the word *gestalt*, which is a German word that refers to a unified whole or a whole shape. While many choral and voice teachers remain focused solely on the larynx during voice change, I advocate the idea that female and male adolescent voice change is truly a whole or gestalt experience, if ever there was one!

Fear of the unknown or the uncontrollable seems to drive much of the perception of adolescent voice change for students and music educators. Although voice change is a complex process, working with changing voices does not have to be a mystery or scary for anyone. Rather, with understanding of the larger process comes a sense of calm and empowerment. So let's do that! Let's fearlessly ponder the gestalt of adolescence as it could relate to voice change. This chapter addresses topics that connect to female and male voice change experiences in some way, including scrutiny, general body growth and coordination, adolescent brain and cognitive development, growth of the hearing mechanism, and emotion. Laryngeal growth and vocal anatomy and physiology (both generally and during adolescent voice change) are discussed at length in chapter 2.

Los! Andiamo! Onwards!

UNDER SCRUTINY

Adolescents are heavily influenced by the invisible audience that watches and judges their every move, every word, and every fashion choice. The mood of the invisible audience depends on the mood of the adolescent; sometimes it is an evil presence that can leave the adolescent feeling insecure and unsure how to act, talk, and think, while other times it can feel gracious and loving.

Beyond the invisible audience, adolescents constantly fight a deficit perspective in the larger world. In *Act Your Age!* Lesko writes,

> A little conscious attention finds adolescents in television sitcoms; in social science, psychology, and therapy; and in news-making discussions of public problems. Typically, teenagers appear in our cultural talk as synonymous with crazed hormones, as delinquents, deficiencies, or clowns, that is, beings not to be taken too seriously. They are most often spoken of with familiarity, sometimes with affection, and regularly with some hostility or displeasure. In these various venues and with decidedly mixed emotions, we talk about "the trouble with teenagers." (2012, p. 1)

In my Internet searches for articles about teens or adolescence, I can easily find a plethora of articles with titles along the lines of "Sorry, Parents: Middle School Is Scientifically the Worst," "How to Stop Your Middle Schooler from Acting So Self-Centered," or "Why Your Grumpy Teenager Doesn't Want to Talk to You." Words such as *surly, tumultuous, miserable, cringe-worthy*, and *worst* pop off the screen all over the place. When I am in search of articles that highlight adolescent intelligence, ability, or compassion, I struggle to find an abundance of sources.

As an advocate for adolescents, I am acutely aware of the glass-is-half-empty mentality that society and pop culture perpetuate about the age group. I am also struck by the unfairness of it all: Adolescents put enormous pressure on themselves to keep the invisible audience happy while they experience physiological, psychological, emotional, and cognitive development that is out of their control while simultaneously fighting expectations of the larger society that they will be horrible and constantly brooding. How does anyone ever make it through adolescence with all of that to battle?

In this book, I encourage readers to check judgment at the door and consider adolescents with compassion and gentleness. What they need most from us as their music educators is kindness, consistency, and empathy so that they can navigate the complex waters leading from childhood to adulthood with as much judgment-free support as we can provide.

PHYSICAL DEVELOPMENT

Hormonal signals from the brain to the gonads (ovaries in females, testes in males) initiate puberty, which is when adolescent bodies mature and become capable of sexual reproduction. Physical signs of puberty include breast development, hair growth under arms and around genitals, the start of menstruation, muscle growth, sex organ growth, voice change, the appearance of acne, and an increase in body odor.

Physical growth and development during adolescence are different for each person. They are sporadic and unpredictable, contributing to issues of clumsiness, awkwardness, and motor skill challenges. (I admit that I find this characteristic of adolescents incredibly endearing.) Sometimes different body parts even grow at different rates, in a phenomenon known as asynchronicity. Sporadic and quick body growth might lead some adolescents to carry themselves with poor posture. Stooping down or slouching helps hide how tall you might be; slouching and curving the shoulders forward are helpful when wanting to hide breast development. A slumped stature is also a way to deflect attention from oneself and put out a "leave me alone" vibe, especially if someone is feeling self-conscious about their body. Many adolescents struggle with body image as a result of being underweight or overweight.

Adolescents have to relearn the map of their body as they re-coordinate movement of limbs and appendages. They may experience growing pains in their legs and arms that leave them in aching pain and there's not much they can do about it. In addition, physical size sometimes results in incorrect assumptions about an adolescent's ability level, attention span, or intelligence level. Bigger adolescents are not always the most mature, worldly, or intelligent students; their voices have not necessarily matured. Smaller adolescents are not always immature or unintelligent; their voices are not necessarily childlike.

Adolescents have *so* much happening to their bodies that is outside of their control, it's quite remarkable. Our work as choral educators allows us to support physical growth and the overall well-being of individual adolescent singers. We can provide opportunities for students to better understand their larger body map and to regain coordination as they grow (i.e., simple movement exercises, walking on the beat in place, simple choreography, and stretching activities). Equipped with a clearer understanding of their body, adolescents may feel more confident and capable during physical changes, which will only assist them in their work as musicians.

HORMONES

Hormones trigger the start of puberty and initiate physiological changes in adolescents. According to the neuroscientist Frances E. Jensen, scientists have known for years *how* hormones work but have only recently discovered *why* they operate the way they do. She writes,

> Because sex hormones are present at birth, they essentially hibernate for more than a decade. What, then, triggers them to begin puberty? A few years ago, researchers discovered that puberty is initiated by what appears to be a game of hormonal dominoes, which begins with a gene producing a single protein, named kisspeptin, in the hypothalamus, the part of the brain that regulates metabolism. When that protein connects with, or "kisses," receptors on another gene, it eventually triggers the pituitary gland to release its storage of hormones. These surges of testosterone, estrogen, and progesterone in turn activate the testes and ovaries. (Jensen, 2015, p. 21)

I find it fascinating how a simple event between two genes leads to such a massive chain reaction of physiological development. The potency and effects of this hormonal chain reaction, however, are largely (and problematically) blamed for adolescent demeanor. Jensen states:

> Hormones have gotten a bad rap with parents and educators, who tend to blame them for everything that goes wrong with teenagers. I always thought the

> expression "raging hormones" made it seem as though these kids had taken a wicked potion or cocktail that made them act with wild disregard for anyone and anything. But we are truly blaming the messenger when we cite hormones as the culprit. Think about it: When your three-year-old has a temper tantrum, do you blame it on raging hormones? Of course not. We know, simply, that three-year-olds haven't yet figured out how to control themselves. In some ways, that's true of teenagers as well. And when it comes to hormones, the most important thing to remember is that the teenage brain is "seeing" these hormones for the first time. Because of that, the brain hasn't yet figured out how to modulate the body's response to this new influx of chemicals. (pp. 19–20)

Jensen goes on to explain that teenagers actually do not have higher hormone levels than do young adults; they simply react differently to hormones. In addition, certain hormones affect adults differently than they do adolescents. For example, the hormone tetrahydropregnenolone is released as a stress response to ease anxiety: In adults, this hormone calms; in adolescents, it has the opposite effect, increasing anxiety. It takes a while for adolescent bodies to regulate hormone production. Side effects from this regulation process can impact daily life in ways adolescents (and their families) never fathomed. In addition to what has been discussed already about the onset of puberty and what is discussed in chapter 2 with regard to the influence of hormones on the changing voice, I would like to share my personal experiences as a young adolescent navigating new hormone surges.

My middle school days weren't always great, but my overall experience was pretty good. One thing that stands out from my adolescent years was the way my body violently reacted to the start of puberty. I had very little control over how I physically felt for much of middle school. The fluctuation of hormones in my body happened in such a way that I threw up *every day* before school for an entire year during my seventh and eighth grade school years. No matter what I did, no matter what doctors recommended, no matter how hard I tried to fend it off—including standing on the porch of my Michigan home in the dead of winter with no coat, trying to shiver the nausea away—I threw up every day for a year. Then one day it just stopped.

I also experienced debilitating migraines every 28 days (which is the length of a typical menstrual cycle) for the first few years of puberty. My migraines started in the morning after I got on the school bus and left me unable to see for most of a day owing to a blinding visual aura; I was also violently ill for that entire day. My wonderful mother kept track of the days and figured out the pattern without telling me. She would wait by the phone after I got on the bus on the designated migraine day, hoping that

I wouldn't call her to come get me after I arrived at school, but for a very long time I always did. I also experienced excruciatingly painful abdominal cramps that were once believed to be ovarian cysts, sometimes making it too painful for me to walk. All medical tests came back inconclusive, and at some point that pain just stopped.

Experiences like these gave me trouble and fostered great fear of going to school and being sick, eating in restaurants and getting sick, going on vacation and getting sick, spending the night at a friend's house and being sick, and so on. It became hard to do anything without being afraid of becoming ill, which also included fear of guilt about the possibility of becoming ill and ruining everyone else's fun time. It was a vicious few years. I remember asking my dad at one point if I was going to die—not a question you want to entertain as an adolescent. My body continued to grow and change, and eventually the issues ceased as I outgrew them.

Other than a few select people, no one knew that all of this was going on while I attended school every day. My parents were incredibly kind and compassionate to me during those years. Because I had choir first thing in the morning in middle school and often wasn't feeling very well at that hour, my choir teacher, Deb McMartin-Finkel, also had the inside information. She was sweet and occasionally checked in with me in the mornings at school. It was nice to have allies at home and at school during this time of great frustration. The kindness and the "you are not weird" vibes from my family and my music teacher (and a few other amazing adults at my school, such as Ms. Sandstrom) during such upsetting circumstances greatly influenced who I am today and my interactions with adolescents. We never really know the entire story of what our students are experiencing during puberty and, as they navigate external physiological growth, they may also be suffering from hormonal changes and challenges affecting them in ways we cannot perceive. Overt kindness and compassion can make a huge difference to all of our adolescent students, but especially those fighting internal, unseen battles with their bodies.

THE ADOLESCENT BRAIN

The brain is an incredibly complex and amazing organ comprised of many regions that govern different facets of our being and doing. The psychiatrist Daniel J. Siegel provided a really handy (yes, pun intended) way to picture the basic construction of the brain in his book *Brainstorm: The Power and Purpose of the Teenage Brain* (2015). As our discussion progresses, it may be helpful to refer to this description:

If you fold your thumb into your palm, and then fold the fingers over your thumb, you'll have facing you a useful hand model of the brain. Give it a try right now and let's see how these parts fit together. In this model the area of your fingernails facing you is just behind the face—and the back of your hand is where the back of the brain at the back of your head would be.

The highest part of the brain, represented by your fingers, is just under your scalp within your skull. This is the *cortex* or outer bark of the brain. We think and reflect, perceive and remember, plan and make decisions with our cortex. Awareness comes, in part, from what happens in the cortex, and so self-awareness comes from this cortical region. If you lift your fingers, you'll see below them the thumb, which represents the emotion-generating *limbic area* of the brain. The limbic area is in charge of a lot of things, including what motivates us, how we focus our attention, and how we remember things. Lift the thumb, and you'll find in your palm the lowest and oldest area of the brain, the *brainstem.* This ancient region is involved in keeping us awake or letting us sleep. And it's the part of the brain that can interact with the thumb region above it, the limbic area, to create reactive states of being angry or scared. Since the brainstem and limbic areas are below the cortex, we call these the "subcortical regions." Lift your fingers and put them back over the thumb and palm and you'll see how the cortex literally sits on top of these two subcortical regions.

The brain itself sits atop the spinal cord, represented by your wrist. Input from this neural tube within the backbone, along with other neural inputs from the body and from the body's organs such as the heart and intestines, enables the processes of our organs, muscles, and bones to directly influence the neural firings in the skull itself, neural activity within the subcortical and cortical parts of the brain. Not represented here is the *cerebellum*, which would be just behind the limbic area and plays an important role in balancing the body's motions and also balancing the interaction of our thoughts and feelings. A band of neurons, called the *corpus callosum*, links the left and right sides of the brain to each other and coordinates and balances their activities. (Siegel, 2015, pp. 86–87)

The adolescent brain is important to our work with populations undergoing voice change for two reasons. First, "adolescent brain growth" is often a broad, sweeping explanation used to justify adolescent behaviors and choices, especially those deemed not very desirable (although the bigger picture is just not that simple). Second, as choral educators, we are constantly influencing the adolescent brain whether we realize it or not. The more we recognize our potential to influence, the more good work we can do for our students in many capacities. The following are a few facts related to the adolescent brain, with full acknowledgment that I am barely scratching the surface of all that *could* be discussed. I draw from work by the psychology professor Laurence Steinberg, PhD (author of *Age of Opportunity: Lessons from the New Science of Adolescence*, 2014) and Frances E. Jensen, MD (author of *The Teenage Brain*, 2015), whose research has focused on helping people better understand how the adolescent brain functions.

The human brain reaches adult size at about the age of ten years, so saying that adolescents experience brain *growth* is not really accurate. Rather, the brain *rewires* itself significantly during adolescence, allowing it to become more organized in preparation for adulthood:

> The connectivity of the brain slowly moves from the back of the brain to the front. The very last places to "connect" are the frontal lobes. In fact, the teen brain is only about 80 percent of the way to maturity. That 20 percent gap, where the wiring is the thinnest, is crucial and goes a long way toward explaining why teenagers behave in such puzzling ways—their mood swings, irritability, impulsiveness, and explosiveness; their inability to focus, to follow through, and to connect with adults; and their temptations to use drugs and alcohol and to engage in other risky behavior. When we think of ourselves as civilized, intelligent adults, we really have the frontal and prefrontal parts of the cortex to thank. (Jensen, 2015, p. 37)

All of this brain rewiring takes time, and it can last well into the early twenties. As the brain insulates the new connections within (a process called myelination) to operate more effectively as an adult,

> sometimes a signal from one area of the brain, say fear and stress coming from the amygdala, has trouble linking up with another part of the brain, for instance the front cortex's sense of judgement. For adolescents whose brains are still being wired, this means they sometimes find themselves in dangerous situations, not knowing what they should do next. (Jensen, 2015, p. 60)

In her book Jensen describes intense real-life scenarios of teenagers who made decisions that could have ended very badly. As I read I was struck by minor decisions that students make in our classrooms on a daily basis that, while not potentially life-threatening, make our days as adolescent educators more colorful. Students' decisions are less mystifying when you step back and consider the effects of brain rewiring on logic or judgment. In moments of frustration, asking an adolescent, "What are you thinking?!" is likely not going to be fruitful because adolescents sometimes make choices and decisions not rooted in thinking about the end game and consequences. Rather, they are in the moment and one step logically leads to the next. A favorite example of this thinking-in-the-moment comes from *Diary of a*

Wimpy Kid (2007) by Jeff Kinney. This book is the fictional story of Greg Heffley, who describes his first year of middle school in entries from his journal, which is "not a diary" (p. 1).

> <u>TUESDAY</u>
>
> Today we got our Independent Study assignment, and guess what it is? We have to build a robot. At first everybody kind of freaked out, because we thought we were going to have to build the robot from scratch. But Mr. Darnell told us we don't have to build an actual robot. We just need to come up with ideas for what our robot might look like and what kinds of things it would be able to do.
>
> Then he left the room, and we were on our own. We started brainstorming right away. I wrote down a bunch of ideas on the blackboard: do my homework, do the dishes, make my breakfast, brush my teeth. Everybody was pretty impressed with my ideas, but it was easy to come up with them. All I did was write down the things I hate doing myself.
>
> But a couple of the girls got up to the front of the room, and they had some ideas of their own. They erased my list and drew up their own plan. They wanted to invent a robot that would give you dating advice and have ten types of lip gloss on its fingertips. All of us guys thought this was the stupidest idea we ever heard. So we ended up splitting into two groups, girls and boys. The boys went to the other side of the room while the girls stood around talking.
>
> Now that we had all the serious workers in one place, we got to work. Someone had the idea that you can say your name to the robot and it can say it back to you. But then someone else pointed out that you shouldn't be able to use bad words for your name, because the robot shouldn't be able to curse. So we decided we should come up with a list of all the bad words the robot shouldn't be able to say. We came up with all the regular bad words, but then Ricky Fisher came up with twenty more the rest of us had never even heard before. So Ricky ended up being one of the most valuable contributors on the project.
>
> Right before the bell rang, Mr. Darnell came back in the room to check on our progress. He picked up the piece of paper we were writing on and read it over. To make a long story short, independent study is canceled for the rest of the year. Well, at least it is for us boys. So if the robots in the future are going around with cherry lip gloss for fingers, at least now you know how it all got started. (Kinney, 2007, pp. 146–150)

I love this part of the story because it makes complete sense to me as an adolescent educator: I completely, logically understand how this (hilarious) scenario could play out with no nefarious intent. The line of thinking here is feasible, especially considering that logic wiring in the adolescent brain is still under construction. As choral educators, we can learn a great deal by talking with students to understand their thought processes and how they arrived at their end point. What step logically led to the next? As adults, our initial responses to situations might be frustration and confusion. However, conversations with our students provide insight into how they think and why they make specific choices, and allow us to guide students back on track. Honest dialogue with adolescents can often lead to beneficial and productive outcomes instead of resulting in frustration and consequences.

The adolescent brain is often described as "plastic" during this rewiring period, indicating the malleability or plasticity of the brain during this stage of life; the brain has the unique ability to mold itself. Steinberg notes:

> When we say the brain is plastic, we mean something that is truer to the actual derivation of the word. "Plastic" comes from the Greek word *plastikos*, derived from the verb *plassein*, which means "to mold." A plastic brain is a brain that can be molded—like industrial plastic before it has been hardened into its final shape. In this sense, the word "plastic" is in fact an excellent way to describe the brain at certain points in development, because just as plastic can be transformed from a soft, malleable state into one that is hard and rigid, so too does the brain change from being relatively more moldable to relatively more fixed. The adolescent brain is more like plastic in its soft, pliable form than in the form it takes after it has been allowed to harden. (Steinberg, 2014, p. 23)

According to both Steinberg and Jensen, the adolescent brain is sculpted by *all* experiences, both passive and active. "Before our brain has fully matured, we can be affected, in potentially permanent ways, by *every* experience, whether it's positive or negative" (Steinberg, 2014, p. 27). Because each person experiences life individually and thoughts, feelings, comments, interactions with others, and so on are different for each person, every brain is unique. "Our brains, in essence, are self-built. They not only serve the particular needs and functions of the particular individual, but also are shaped—landscaped if you will—by the individual's particular experiences" (Jensen, 2015, p. 68).

The more adolescents experience something—a specific activity, a happy or fearful emotion, a thought—the more the neural connections in their brains are strengthened and that experience is retained. In music classes, the more adolescents sing particular passages, experience empathy via understandings of text or class discussions, experience fear about a specific note or vocal range, feel joy about accomplishing a task, feel embarrassment about singing because their voice cracked, and so forth, the more neural connections related to those experiences are strengthened in the brain.

We must also consider each student's life story in all of this. When adolescents feel supported, cared for, fed, warmed, clothed, and loved, all of these experiences strengthen connections in their brains, influencing development and serving the needs of the individual. When adolescents feel belittled, neglected, abused, uncertain where food will come from, experience unstable living conditions, or feel unsafe, all of these experiences also strengthen connections in the brain and influence development. What our students encounter and feel stays with them on a biological level, giving us as choral educators prime opportunities to reinforce positive experiences, especially if we have students for more than one academic year. We can provide beneficial experiences for students that may influence or counterbalance some of what they face outside of our classrooms. We are also in a prime position to reinforce successful singing experiences for all of our students, especially during voice change. Scientific research implies that our work as choral educators can be a powerful influence on the ways that our students' brains rewire, both inside and outside our classrooms. *How* we choose to wield that influence is up to each of us.

Electronic Communication and Brain Development

The November 2016 issue of *Time* featured the article "The Kids Are Not All Right" by Susanna Schrobsdorff and focused on anxiety and depression in American teenagers. Among a number of important discussion points, one aspect of the article was particularly poignant: the impact of the hyperconnectedness of adolescents to each other and emotional outcomes of those connections. "It's hard for many adults to understand how much of teenagers' emotional life is lived within the small screens on their phones," Schrobsdorff wrote (p. 47). I have two stories that relate to this matter before returning to brain development.

First, one summer when I was teaching the Illinois Summer Youth Music junior chorus, we learned a song that had silly words about our knowing that we were fabulously good-looking. I asked the singers to be flirtier or to flirt more with an imaginary person as we declared our good looks. At the break, a young man approached me and said, "Dr. Sweet . . . I don't know what you mean by 'flirt' as I only ever text girls." It was a fascinating comment while it was also a bit sad that his only interactions with girls were via his phone.

Second, in the same summer when the youth choir incident took place, I was speaking with one of the camp counselors, who told me that she had been on dorm rounds the previous evening and passed by the recreation room, where most of the middle school campers were gathered at the end of the day. When she walked by the room, it was completely silent. She looked in and saw that all the students were there, sitting in little circles around the room. No one was talking because everyone was looking at their own phone (while sitting in circle formation with friends). The counselor knew they were communicating within each circle because one person would send out something funny to the rest of that circle, everyone would laugh, and then their heads would go back down as they typed responses to each other. No one was actually talking person-to-person. Again, I was completely fascinated.

In the book *The Owner's Manual for Driving Your Adolescent Brain* (2013), the psychologists JoAnn Deak and Terrence Deak (who are related as aunt and nephew) explained how one structure in our brain, the right temporal parietal junction (RTPJ), is "particularly important for developing empathy, a critical ingredient for positive social interactions throughout life" (p. 44). Yet the overabundance of electronic communication in today's world is impacting the way adolescents use their RTPJ and their ability to communicate and demonstrate empathy:

> Recent data suggests that many young people may not be using their RTPJ as much as they could because they spend so much time communicating electronically through digital devices, text messages, or social networks. While scientists are still figuring out how relationships built through technology compare to personal interaction, most believe that person-to-person connection is essential for adolescents to learn effective and appropriate ways of interacting in the world. This is true in other species as well: when contact with other rodents is restricted, even these small creatures fail to develop normal social interactions. These effects are particularly pronounced when social interaction is restricted during adolescence, suggesting that this is a critical/sensitive period for social interaction. You can improve your own chances for healthy social interaction as an adult by ensuring that your interactions with others are not limited to just electronic means such as texting or emailing. (Deak & Deak, 2013, p. 45)

During junior chorus rehearsals at the summer music camp, the middle school students interacted with me and with each other for many hours. They shared thoughts about the music and assumptions about composers' intentions, revealed emotional stories from their own lives, sang together beautifully, and laughed *a lot*. Although the campers chose to communicate with each other outside rehearsal by electronic methods, I know that during our time together working on choral music, we locked down some new RTPJ functionality. I understand that the world we live in is a wired, hyperconnected one and that the adolescent campers were just being themselves in my stories above, but that means that my work—*your work*—as a choral music educator is more crucial than ever to offset adolescents' hyperconnectedness and promote growth of the right temporal parietal junction. We already know that the choral experiences we provide can be rich with person-to-person communication, promotion of empathy and understanding, and shared human experience. But whereas our profession has historically remained focused on *musical* experiences, it is time to more mindfully assume a more active role in the brain development of our adolescent students.

Hearing Development

When starting this book, I attempted to locate research that documented growth of the hearing mechanism in order to better understand hearing changes (i.e., ability to perceive pitches) that seem to occur during puberty. I ultimately sought assistance from my Speech and Hearing Science colleagues at the University of Illinois and audiologists and hearing specialists from around the country, who recommended several research articles that in some way addressed what I was seeking. These articles were *extremely* dense and complex, using an entire vocabulary system outside that of music education. While I will not share all aspects of the research I have read, I am excited to share the crux of this research and suggest implications for our work as choral educators.

More than anything, adolescent hearing development has a great deal to do with the *entire* auditory system. The auditory system is divided into two subsystems. The first subsystem is the peripheral auditory system, which consists of the outer ear, the middle ear, and the inner ear. The second is the central auditory system, which begins with the cochlear nucleus and extends to the primary auditory cortex in the brain. In her article "Development of the Auditory System," the otolaryngology professor Ruth Y. Litovsky writes,

> Generally, the auditory system serves the role of constructing a perceptual space that extracts information from objects (animate and inanimate), groups together some objects, and segregates sounds from one another. In other words,

the auditory system engages in an analysis of the auditory world, so that the listener can accomplish the goal of communication and learning. (Litovsky, 2015, p. 55)

Litovsky briefly discusses physiological growth of the first subsystem, acknowledging that changes occur within this subsystem during childhood and early adolescence:

> The ear is responsible for the initial encoding of acoustic input. The functional status of the ear has been studied using numerous investigational and clinical tools. Anatomic studies suggest that numerous changes occur after full-term birth. For example, the anatomy of the human ear canal continues to mature; in infants the canal is shorter and straighter than it is in adults (Northern & Downs, 1984). Another example is the increase in ear canal diameter and length during the first 2 years of life (Keefe, Bulen, Arehart, & Burns, 1993). Finally, even more prolonged is the development of the middle-ear cavity volume, which extends into the late teenage years, which is likely to influence the mechanics involved in middle-ear function (Eby & Nadol, 1986). The postnatal maturation of the external and middle ear is important to note, because they can have substantial effects on how sounds are absorbed, processed, filtered, and transmitted to the auditory system. (pp. 2–3)

It could be inferred from Dr. Litovsky's writings that physiological growth of the components of the outer, middle, and inner ear during late childhood and early adolescence could influence the hearing function and pitch perceptions of adolescents in choral and singing contexts. For those of us who work with adolescent singers this seems logical, because middle-level singers often experience challenges in hearing, determining, and distinguishing various pitches. Whereas our work with adolescent singers does involve that first subsystem, it may more significantly involve the auditory cortex of the second subsystem (beginning with the cochlear nucleus and extending to the primary auditory cortex in the brain) as our students physically grow during adolescence—which is why I placed this discussion about hearing in the section of this chapter about the adolescent brain. The following are a few highlights from articles provided to me by the aforementioned audiologists that connect adolescent hearing with brain function.

The cognitive neuroscientist Elyse S. Sussman conducted the research described in "Attention Matters: Pitch vs. Pattern Processing in Adolescence" in which she examined the idea of attention as something that is adaptive. She wrote,

> More sensory information reaches us that [*sic*] we can possibly deal with. One of the goals of attention is to limit the amount of information we perceive. When we choose to attend to certain parts of the sensory input it changes our experience of the environment. (2013, p. 1)

Can adolescents (as listeners) focus their attention on different aspects of sounds? Specifically, how well are adolescents able to focus their listening on individual pitches, a pattern of sounds, or no sound at all?

For Sussman's study, ten adolescents (six male, four female, ranging in ages from 13 to 17 years) listened to tone sequences that required three ways of attentive listening: Attend-Pitch, Attend-Pattern, and Attend-Video. During the Attend-Pitch condition, participants "were instructed to listen to the three different pitches of the tones and press the response key when they heard the rarely occurring, lowest-pitched tone" (p. 3). During the Attend-Pattern condition, participants "were instructed that there was a five-tone repeating pattern of tones in the sequence and to press the response key when they detected a different pattern that occurred rarely" (p. 3). And last, in the Attend-Video condition, "participants were told that they would hear sounds in their ears, to ignore the sounds and watch the captioned video of their choosing" (p. 3).

What Sussman found was that each way of listening elicited different neural responses in the participants' brains:

> These results thus demonstrate that selective attention alters neural activity, adapting the neural response to the pertinent elements of the input required for performing a task: in this case, adapting to a five-tone standard in one condition and to single-tone standard in the other. (p. 6)

She went on to state that the ability to selectively focus on a specific sound and ignore irrelevant sounds in the environment concerns changes in neurophysiologic response and is attributed to the ability to control one's attention, noting, "Overall, the results show, in adolescence [*sic*] as in adults, that attention plays an important role in modulating neural activity to facilitate performance, adjusting the time scale of adaption dependent upon task goals" (p. 7).

For the world of choral music, Sussman's research implies that our adolescent singers have the ability to listen to individual pitches as well as patterns of pitches, but such tasks require focused attention plus neural activity. And though their brains have the ability to switch between actively focusing on individual pitches and focusing on a pattern, development of required adjustments in the brain between tasks can take time.

She advised that we plan our time scale accordingly if we have a specific goal in mind. In addition, the greater the extraneous noise during such processes, the longer it may take to accomplish specific goals. Sussman's research supports practicing often in short, focused durations, not ongoing and belabored sessions; intentional quiet in the chorus room during key moments will also be helpful. This study leads me to rethink the way we go about other singing activities as well, such as asking adolescent singers to find their starting pitch within the notes of a different vocal line. Such a request requires them not only to focus on an individual note but also to pull it out from among a pattern of notes, and according to Sussman's research, such an activity requires the brain to switch gears mid-activity, as the student listens to a pattern and an individual pitch. Accomplishing this task may take more time than we would like to give, but this study supports patient and repeated efforts and indicates that success is possible.

In the article "Continued Maturation of Auditory Brainstem Function During Adolescence: A Longitudinal Approach," six scientists (a mixture of neuroscientists and otolaryngologists) described tracking the auditory brainstem development of 74 adolescents for four years, from age 14 to age 17 (Krizman et al., 2015). They did this by examining the adolescents' subcortical evoked response (the subcortical area is the "tucked thumb" area of the hand model of the brain discussed earlier). Subcortical responses were monitored by connecting the adolescents to a range of sensors and having them watch a movie of their choice. The researchers were not concerned with how the adolescents' hearing mechanisms interacted with the sounds of the movie, but rather with how their auditory brainstem interpreted the sounds they heard. Ultimately, the researchers found that changes to the auditory brainstem do not stop altogether at about age two, as previously believed, but continue to take place between the ages of 14 and 17. And furthermore:

> In addition to arguing for a reevaluation of the maturational time course of the auditory brainstem, our results also suggest that enriched or diminished experiences later in childhood can have a larger effect on auditory function than previously believed (Skoe & Kraus, 2013; Tierney, Krizman, Skoe, Johnston, & Krause, 2013). Given the assumption that plasticity of the nervous system declines dramatically beyond mid-childhood, previous studies of the auditory system have suggested an age of 7–10 years as the closing of a heightened period of malleability in response to experience. It has therefore been argued that exposure to certain experiences such as music or second-language learning must

> begin early in life for a child to realize the full potential of those skills (Asher & Garcia, 1969; Watanabe et al., 2007). That the auditory brainstem has not fully matured until the end of adolescence suggests that auditory enrichment begun later in childhood (e.g., ~14 years) could still lead to sizeable enhancements in auditory processing and alter developmental profiles. (p. 2353)

When considered from the viewpoint of choral music education, this scientific discovery supports students who want to begin singing "later in childhood" (which, according to the researchers' age determination, is in early adolescence) because their brains are still primed and ready to learn new musical skills. It also supports my hunch that middle-school singers are learning to hear in new ways at the same time their voices are changing. This means that students with what seems to be a one- or two-note range should be treated with even more patience because (a) their vocal mechanism is not coordinated enough to formulate multiple pitches at the moment and (b) their auditory cortex is also learning to determine and understand the new sounds they are attempting to sing. One more detail to note from this study is that as adolescents physically grow during puberty, their head size and skull thickness increase. While this growth has been shown to affect "auditory-evoked potentials" (Krizman et al., 2015, p. 2354), the researchers reported that this is a relatively minor detail in normal adolescent development. Therefore, head size and skull thickness are not likely factors for us to consider with regard to our adolescent musicians matching pitch in middle-school choir.

Three of the neuroscientists discussed above, Adam T. Tierney, Jennifer Krizman, and Nina Kraus, conducted a separate study to learn more about how experiences interact with the developmental plasticity (the changes in neural connections during development) of the brain during adolescence. According to their article "Music Training Alters the Course of Adolescent Auditory Development," they followed two groups of high school students, one engaged in a school music ensemble and the other engaged in Junior Reserve Officers' Training Corps. Data were collected just before the students began high school and again four years later, during their last year of high school. Although the full report was written for a brain-research audience (please see the full report for the scientific details), I am pleased to share some of the reported findings that relate to discussion of voice change in this book.

First, Tierney, Krizman, and Kraus clearly acknowledged that the creation of new neural pathways, also referred to as synaptic density, slows down as we get older, as early as young adulthood. This is why it is more challenging for us to learn a second language as we get older than it is for young children; the brain forms new nerve synapses easily when we are younger and not so much as we age. The results of this study suggest, however, that while "response consistency peaks in childhood (~8–11 y of age), declining steadily until young adulthood[,] . . . this adolescent decline is mitigated by in-school music lessons" (Tierney, Krizman, & Kraus, 2015, p. 10064). The researchers also reported that "music training may maintain heightened synaptic density within the auditory system to enable the learning and performance of challenging auditory tasks" (p. 10064).

Therefore, involvement in music classes, even as late as high school, can slow the decline of synapsis formation in the brain-related portions of students' auditory system (again, the body system responsible for the sense of hearing). And, in fact, these researchers believe that taking music classes actually encourages a significant increase in the creation of new synapses (called synaptogenesis) in the brain-related portions of the auditory system "much as songbirds show seasonal increases in synaptogenesis that coincide with the onset of the preferential period for learning new songs" (p. 10064). These findings are encouraging for all music educators, as they provide scientific evidence for biological benefits from involvement in music classes that could: positively impact students for the rest of their lives; assist in continued advocacy efforts for the larger music education profession; and offer insight on a larger potential for our work as choral educators.

Teaching adolescents during voice change means that we are working with humans during a time of major brain rewiring. In our choral education programs, a myriad of experiences—be they musical, emotional, social, cognitive, or psychological—contribute to this rewiring. Sometimes the experiences we provide in music classes correlate with influences from home, other classes, and social contexts; sometimes they are in opposition. Sometimes the reinforcement of this wiring in our choral classrooms is intentional, and sometimes it is not. The bottom line is that everything our adolescent students experience during their time with us influences their brain in some way during its rewiring process on the way to adulthood.

Research indicates that adolescents think and process differently than adults because of how their brains are wired, so expecting them to think and act and reason like adults is unrealistic. It is also unrealistic as generation gaps between us and our young students widen. I believe that the choral music education profession would benefit from embracing increased knowledge about adolescent brain development as well as a deeper understanding that patience and time are important tools in teaching adolescent singers because of the many biological implications of puberty. More holistic considerations will only lead us to be more strategic, realistic, patient, positive, and productive music educators, especially when working with adolescent students.

EMOTION

Voice change can be a very personal and emotional experience for adolescents, made more complex by individual personalities, severity of voice change symptoms, length of time during which students experience vocal challenges, expectations of social circles, the culture of the music classroom, and family context. Scrutiny by the "invisible audience" may heighten emotional reactions to vocal challenges or frustrations. There is much more to come in the following chapters about emotion and voice change specifically, but this is a good place to address more general emotional considerations of adolescents.

When my daughter was three, she would ask me, "Momma, are you happy or sad?" Sometimes I could respond one way or the other, but most often she would ask me in moments when I felt entirely different emotions such as frustration—which I do not define as either happy or sad—or while crying during a movie because I was moved to tears (usually during *Coco* or the end of *Paddington 2*). I could not describe myself as feeling happy or sad, but rather *something else*. This confused her because she did not understand why I could not be either one or the other, happy or sad; she did not yet understand that there are other options.

As children enter adolescence they begin to experience emotions beyond the standard fare of happy, sad, angry, or afraid and often do not understand how to process these new emotions, especially those that catch them off guard. Adolescents in our music classes are likely exploring new emotional territory at home and at school as they become adults. To complicate matters, they may also be experiencing new emotions via social media, websites, chat rooms, so forth. As Schrobsdorff noted in "The Kids Are Not All Right" (2016):

> Phoebe Gariepy, a 17-year old in Arundel, Maine, describes following on Instagram a girl in Los Angeles whom she'd never met because she liked the photos she posted. Then the girl stopped posting. Phoebe later heard she'd been kidnapped and was found on the side of a road, dead. "I started bawling, and

I didn't even know this girl," says Phoebe. "I felt really extremely connected to that situation even though it was in L.A."

That hyperconnectedness now extends everywhere, engulfing even rural teens in a national thicket of Internet drama. Daniel Champer, the director of school-based services for Intermountain in Helena, Mont., says the one word he'd use to describe the kids in his state is *overexposed*. (pp. 47–48)

All of this makes our jobs as educators more complex, particularly in the context of choral music, which is, by its very nature, an emotional medium.

One of my most favorite portrayals of the complexity of adolescent emotion (and the start of adolescence in general) is the Disney-Pixar movie *Inside Out* (Docter, Lasseter, & Stanton, 2015). At the beginning of this story, Riley celebrates her 11th birthday and also moves from Minnesota to San Francisco with her mom and dad. It is a challenging experience for Riley for a number of reasons, but you should watch the whole movie to get the full story. Throughout the movie, Riley's memories (stored in her head) are represented by objects that look like marbles, each of which is a different color to signify the emotion associated with that memory: red marbles represent anger; yellow marbles, joy; green marbles, disgust; blue marbles, sadness; and purple marbles, fear. Each memory is one solid color at the beginning of the movie because Riley's emotional experiences are distinguished the same way my daughter categorized them in her question to me: happy or sad.

At the end of the movie the marbles are no longer one solid color, but multicolored, meaning that Riley's experiences and emotions are growing more complex. For Riley, a moment can be both joyful and scary, both sad and disgusting, both angry and joyful, and so on. The entire concept of *Inside Out* is beautiful, and it is a wonderful portrayal of one girl's journey into adolescence. It is a movie that I recommend to all people working with this age group.

As adolescents navigate increasingly more adult experiences they encounter new emotions and are often unsure how to interpret them or what to do with them. I can remember crying in my middle school counselor's office for an hour in seventh grade, saying, "I'm not even sure why I'm crying! I'm not even sure why I'm crying!" again and again. New emotional experiences can trigger a student to think, "I've never felt this emotion before," quickly leading to "No one has felt this emotion before," which swiftly leads to "No one understands how I am feeling so no one understands *me*." It could be that the adolescent has fallen in love for the first time or has been betrayed by their closest friend for the first time. Regardless of the circumstances, when adolescents perceive that they are alone in their emotions, they unintentionally complicate matters by adding feelings of isolation to the mix; this is especially the case with sad or hurt feelings.

Choral music can be extremely emotional, especially with the interplay between text and music, and our adolescent singers will often express emotion while singing without any intervention on our part. However, part of our work as choral music educators is to intentionally foster emotional connections between the student and the music, between the student and the rest of the choir, and between the student and the larger society. These sorts of connections can come from class discussions, individual journals, composition projects, "this is my life soundtrack" projects, a class book club, community outreach and service, and more. There is no limit to the number of possibilities we can set up in order for our students to experience different emotions.

Experiencing emotions and expressing them are separate things. I have found that asking adolescents to describe with words how they feel about something can be really tricky because they do not always have the vocabulary to articulate such things. On the contrary, if I asked an adolescent to play for me a piece of music or a recording that represents how they feel about something, they would *nail it* immediately. Adolescents have intelligent and insightful thoughts and feelings, but limited strategies to express themselves can keep the ideas and emotions locked inside the student. So while providing opportunities for students to undertake new experiences is important, so is providing varied ways for them to digest their experiences, interpret them, build vocabulary, try different methods to express emotions felt during those experiences, and develop understanding of how to replicate (or avoid) them. Emotion is part and parcel of our work as choral educators, especially those who work with adolescents, and it can be both wonderful and challenging. But I think it might be my favorite aspect of the age group.

Before leaving this discussion of adolescent emotion, I would like to gently remind you that, as choral music educators, you are not licensed, trained counselors or mental health professionals. It is wonderful to be a supportive presence for your students, but you do not have the training to most effectively navigate some of the emotional situations that come your way. If a student seems to be in crisis, stay with them, support them, be with them, hold their hand as you walk them down to the school counselor or administration office. Help your student by requesting help from the people in your building who have both training and access to resources to best help adolescents in crisis. Adolescent counselors are some of the most amazing people I have ever met and their work is incredibly important, especially in combination with that of choral educators.

DIGEST

As a milestone in human development, puberty is quite dramatic, involving a rapid transformation of anatomy, physiology, and behavior. Other than pregnancy, it is probably the most abrupt and encompassing developmental transition that human beings undergo between birth and death.

P. T. Ellison & M. W. Reiches

The goal of this chapter was to provide readers with a gestalt perspective of adolescence (and adolescents) before we launch into more focused discussion of the changing voice. Adolescence is complex and multifaceted, and the way adolescents navigate this time of life greatly influences the way they will think and feel and do as adults. We have a role to play in the process as choral music educators, making the world a bit more bearable for the students in our classes and—as a result of all our good efforts—making the larger world a bit more bearable, too. I worry that many choral educators do not consider the overall student. If we only work with adolescent *voices* and do not consider physical development, the brain, hormones, emotions, and the invisible audience, we are not fulfilling our full charge as choral music educators. Only after we consider the larger components of adolescence and then consider the individual students in our choral programs are we best equipped to choose music, exercises, and experiences that best suit the unique needs of the students in our programs.

Comedian Eddie Izzard included a segment on puberty in his edgy, breakthrough stand-up comedy show, *Dressed to Kill*, which first aired in 1999. His description of the completely topsy-turvy nature of adolescence, the sheer lack of control during most of it, is absolutely spot on. In addition, he weaves voice change into the conversation in a very humorous manner. What follows is a transcript of this portion of his comedy show; be forewarned that it is a bit raunchy at moments, but funny and full of truth.

<begin transcript>

I played kiss-chase with the girls. Tag a girl and she has to kiss you; kind of sexy. But then puberty came and *destroyed* my confidence. It *destroyed* my *everything*. Which I think is part of the thing that causes these kids to go off and commit murder [in reference to an earlier part of the show when he discusses gun violence] because it *is* such a *hell of a gear change*.

Think about it. Because before puberty, girls and boys are going (*making a face like he is disgusted*) "Girls . . . *blech!*" "Boys . . . *blech*!" But then it gets to puberty and it's all (*making a seductive face*) "Girls . . . *ooo! Ahh!*" or "Boys . . . *ooo! Ahh!*" or whatever sexual preference you're going. And you start thinking, "God, I want to get off with some of these people. I'd better look my *best*! And then Mother Nature says, "*NO!* You are going to look *the worst* you've ever looked in your *life!*" (*audience laughing loudly as he looks all around and up and down at his body*) "Hold on! Where did I get all *this* from?!"

We repulse ourselves! I used to look in the mirror and say, "Well, *I'm* not going to shag me, that's for certain!" (*audience laughing*) 'Cause that's what narcissism is all about (*talking in a very suave voice*) is looking in the mirror and going, "Ahh . . . I'd like to have sex with myself!" You know, it's all sort of a self-attraction thing. *And then the acne thing*. And you look at yourself and you go (*with a repulsed voice*), "Ugh. *No way*."

And parents should tell you the facts of puberty! (*talking, like a parent to a child*) "Look, your hair is going to go greasy, your face will become a general plague area. Here's a book on the Black Death. Tufts of hair will grow on your chin . . . not in a sexy, stubble way, but in a continuing plague theme. Down here (*indicating his groin area*)--I'm not even going to *talk* about that!"

And it's over months and years. Puberty is *over months and years*. It should be *one day*. Get the *fucker over with*. Go into school, (*talking in a high-pitched voice*) "Sorry! I don't know why I was late!" By the time you go home, (*talking in a low-pitched voice*) "Right. I'm going home to get a job with a drill."

And that one day at school will be weird: (*high voice*) "Sorry, I don't (*low voice*) know the answer to that question." (*high voice*) "Excuse me, can I be excused? (*low voice*) I seem to have the plague."

And then I had to chat up girls and I've never used my vocal ability to chat up girls. And when your voice is breaking it's very hard saying, (*low voice*) "Susan, I really (*high voice*) kind of (*low voice*) fancy you. I saw you on the (*high voice*) playground."

I had to chat up girls and I'd only tagged them before and I didn't have the verbal power to say, "Susan, I saw you in the classroom today as the sun came from behind the clouds and a burst of brilliant light caught your hair. It was haloed in front of me. You turned your eyes, flashed fire into my soul. I immediately read the words of Dostoyevsky and Karl Marx and in the words of Albert Schweitzer . . . I . . . *fancy you*." (*audience laughing*)

But no! At 13, you're just going (*with a goofy, love-stricken look on his face*) "Hello Sue! I've . . . I've got legs!" (*long pause as he pounds the tops of his thighs with fists for a moment*) "Do you . . . do you . . . like . . . *bread?* I've got French loaf!" (*Then makes a swinging motion with him arm, as if to hit Sue with his loaf of bread and then runs away laughing*) "Bye! I love you!"

<end transcription>

I love this monologue because it rings true for many reasons. The messiness, the unpredictability, the surprise of puberty—he gets it. Each time I listen to it, I am profoundly struck by the line "[puberty] destroyed my everything." I think that is a very honest and, for many, truthful statement about adolescence. Few things are moving or working or predictably playing out as they used to or as they might have been imagined: not the body, not the voice, not the independence, not the identity, not the way of thinking. Puberty and physical change can turn life upside down in many unexpected ways. *Especially* because of all of this, our work as music educators has the potential to be extremely important, meaningful, and long-lasting for adolescents.

As we move forward in this book to focus more intently on adolescent voice change, I encourage you to carry forth the ideas from this chapter as you consider voice change to be a full-self experience. If you are wary of working with changing voices, I urge you to set your fears and feelings of discomfort aside and be open to all of the discussion yet to come. Most important, keep in mind your potential to be a powerful advocate for your adolescent students as well as a very important source of support.

"What you do makes a difference, and you have to decide what kind of difference you want to make." (Jane Goodall, Primatologist)

CHAPTER 2
Anatomy and Physiology

The voice is not a mysterious glowing orb as Ariel's voice is portrayed in Disney's *The Little Mermaid*. Rather, it is produced by a small, complex, and important organ in our body that can be understood, developed, and damaged. Adolescents tend not to have a basic understanding of how the voice is produced, let alone what happens during voice change. This lack of understanding can make the entire experience of voice change scary, confusing, and frustrating. But one thing is certain: knowledge can be extremely powerful. The more adolescent singers understand about vocal anatomy and physiology, the less scary voice change can be, and the more likely they are to persevere through challenges and continue singing.

In her book *Singing and Teaching Singing: A Holistic Approach to Classical Voice*, Janice Chapman notes:

> The understanding of vocal anatomy and physiology is even more important when working with the developing singer, who often has to build his or her instrument simultaneously while learning how to play it. For example, a music student learning the clarinet arrives at college with an instrument one can see, touch, and manipulate. No one expects the student to build the clarinet first. A singer cannot see their voice, has only limited sensation of the instrument, and is strongly reliant on auditory perception, which must be educated over time. In the 21st century, I believe that a very important part of a singing teacher's duty is to inform students about their instrument and how it works. (2012, p. 9)

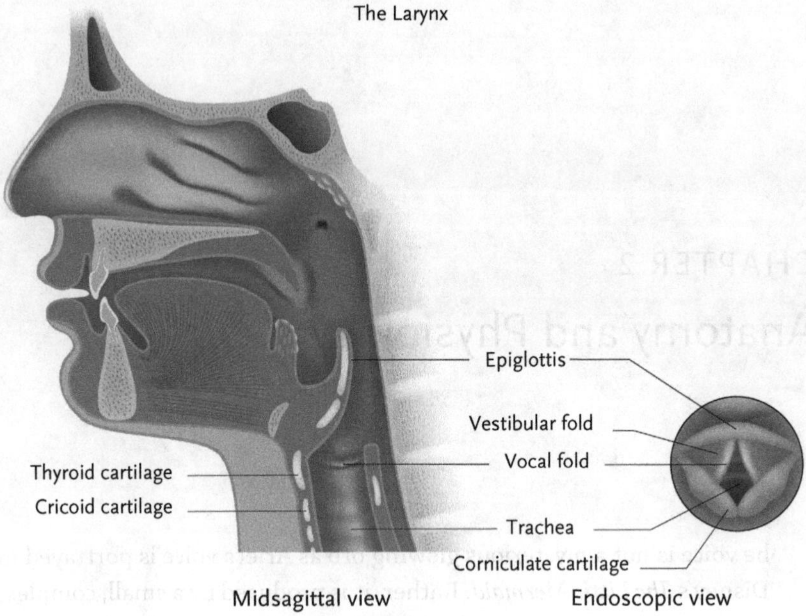

Figure 2.1. The larynx, midsagittal and endoscopic views. (www.Shutterstock.com [120863443].)

Recurring discussions of vocal anatomy, function, and physiological changes during voice change only empower adolescent singers throughout the process. Such conversations also reveal that what is often mistaken as an easy instrument (or not considered an instrument at all) is actually quite complex and extraordinary. Part of the mystery and challenge of the voice is that there are no visuals to reference when using the instrument, no buttons to push or slides to move. The ability to reference posters, images, models, or videos of the larynx and its parts (see figures 2.1 and 2.6), the respiratory system (see figure 2.2), the digestive system (see figure 2.3), and the skeletal system (see figure 2.4) is important in students' transforming mystery and misunderstanding to fact.

The key to using such teaching aids is that they must be explained and referenced on a regular basis so that students truly understand the concepts and terminology, as well as *why* you are sharing this information. As explored in chapter 1, the adolescent brain is much more likely to hardwire information about vocal anatomy and physiology if it is repeated over time. In addition, as students progress through voice change they will focus on different aspects of the information depending on where they are in the process. Students with unchanged voices may

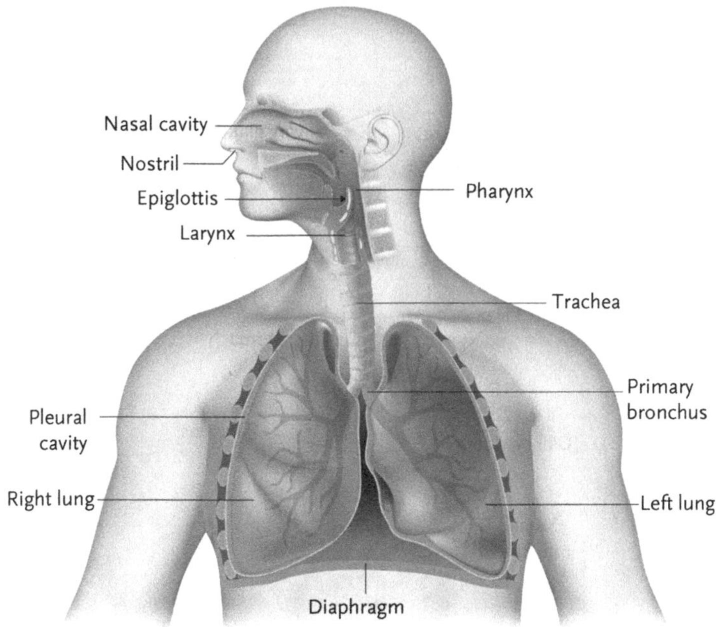

Figure 2.2. The respiratory system. (www.Shutterstock.com [228843244].)

understand the basics of your conversation about vocal anatomy and physiology but might not care much about voice change because they are not yet experiencing any of it. When they begin or are in the midst of voice change, suddenly parts of the conversation seem much more pertinent to their current experiences, and their level of attention and interest will likely increase.

PREVENTING MISUNDERSTANDING

Frequent discussions of anatomy and physiology help dispel myths and prevent misunderstandings about how the voice and body function. For example, I have had the following exchange with middle-level singers on multiple occasions:

ME: It is important to drink lots of water in preparation for our concert. Why?

ADOLESCENT SINGER: Because the water will keep your vocal folds wet.

ME: What do you mean?

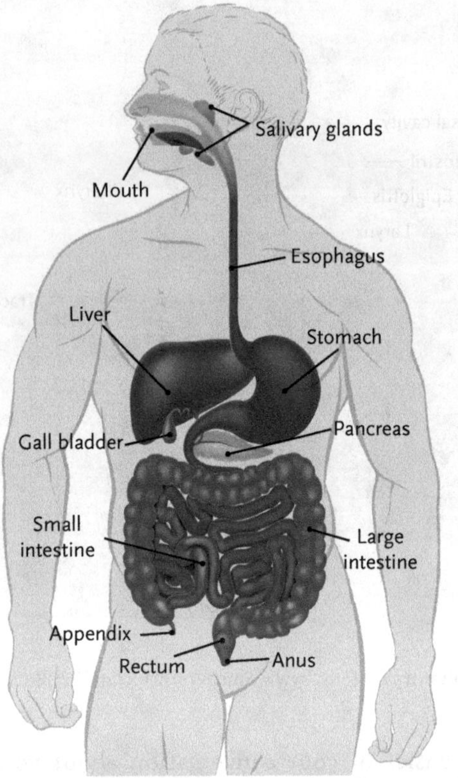

Figure 2.3. The digestive system. (www.Shutterstock.com [367631687].)

> ADOLESCENT SINGER: When I swallow, the water will go over my vocal folds and keep them wet.
>
> ME: Actually, if your vocal folds are wet, that's really *bad* because that means that you are drowning.

Not only do students need to understand general differences between the location and function of the trachea and the esophagus, we need to make it clear *why* what we are discussing matters for singers. Rather than just telling adolescent singers, "Drink lots of water before the concert," our job involves teaching students that drinking water (or other hydrating liquids) hydrates our body and thins out mucus, which in turn keeps our larynx lubricated in much the same way oil works in a car engine. In addition, there is a general belief in the world of speech pathology that our body will hydrate our primary organs first and secondary organs second. Primary organs include the heart, lungs, and brain; the larynx is a secondary organ. When hydrating, we need to take in enough water to supply our primary

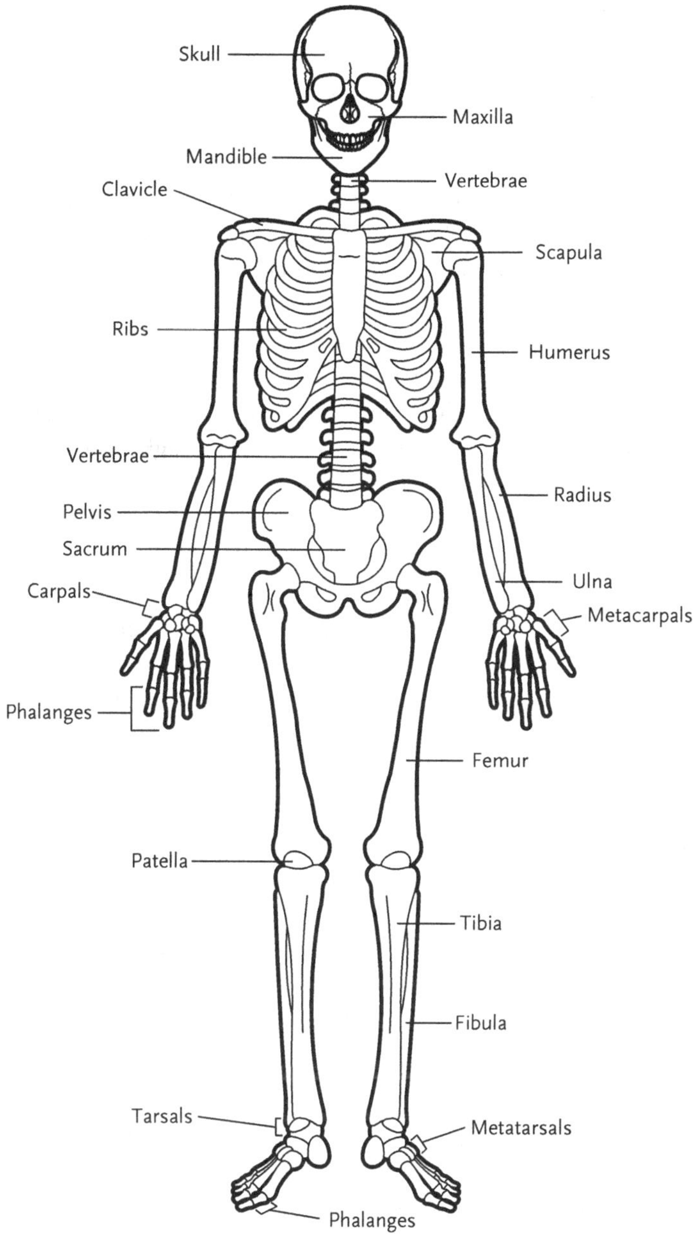

Figure 2.4. The skeletal system. (www.Shutterstock.com [500904814].)

organs and then take care of the larynx. Hydration of the vocal mechanism is discussed at length in the book *The Owner's Manual to the Voice: A Guide for Singers and Other Professional Voice Users* (Gates, Forrest, & Obert, 2013), including information about how some tissue layers benefit from hydration right away and other tissues take longer to receive benefits. So, gulping a bottle of water 20 minutes before a concert is not going to be as beneficial for singers as planning ahead for hydration. The bottom line is that discussions of physiology and the science behind what we do empower our singers and further validate our instrument, as well as head off misunderstandings from the beginning.

With regard to other body systems, understanding that the spine is shaped like the letter *S* clears up the misconception that standing up straight means that the spine will actually be straight; spines are not designed that way so we can move and twist and bend. Instead, have students aim for standing tall (rather than straight) to ensure a long, balanced back. A key element to stance is the skull and its relationship with the spine. The human head, which weighs approximately ten pounds, does not connect to the spine at the back of the skull, and when we are tall and aligned, the skull balances on top of our spine. I find that I can feel a physical difference when my skull is in balance because it feels as if it is just there, easy like a Sunday morning, with no effort to hold it in place. When the head is tipped forward or backward (even just slightly), other parts of our body have to engage to hold the head in place, such as the neck, back, chest, and shoulder muscles. Over time, tension can arise from the unnecessary overworking of these other body parts and contribute to issues of vocal fatigue, loss of vocal stamina, discomfort, or pain.

Earlier in my career, I would run down all the various body parts with my singers: chin parallel to the floor, sternum lifted, shoulders relaxed, hips and feet aligned . . . it was exhausting and my students did not understand *why* this mattered. As I have learned more about body function and mapping, I have found that scientific explanations encourage proper physical stance with adolescent singers (or singers of any age, actually) and provide watertight logic for why we are requesting such stance from our singers. Now I simply ask everyone to stand tall and balance their head on their spine because we have had conversations about spine shape, skull weight, and so on, and my singers understand *why* I am making this request.

Further examples: understanding the basics of the skeletal system increases awareness of the rib cage in the breathing process and why our shoulders should not move when we fill with air. Understanding the basics of the respiratory system promotes awareness of lung expansion all around the body; students more easily notice how the lungs move on the front, sides, and back of the body when they breathe. They also understand the real role of the diaphragm in breathing and singing (that it is a skeletal muscle and most of the time operates involuntarily). Understanding the basics of the digestive system and acknowledging all of our guts helps students appreciate why our bellies go out when we fill with air; it is a displacement consequence and not about body weight or shape. And so on.

Stage fright and performance anxiety manifest in the physiology of the body as hormone levels change when stress begins, triggering a chain reaction of physiological symptoms, all of which can be explained by responses that are hard-wired into us from centuries ago when we might have had to outrun a tiger that wants to eat us for dinner. It's fight or flight, and there is not a lot that we can do about the onset. Those butterflies in your stomach before a performance is your body sending your blood to your limbs so you can outrun that tiger. Your increased heart rate is your body preparing to outrun that tiger. Dry mouth is your body conserving moisture for your primary organs so you can outrun that tiger. Understanding what is physiologically happening and why removes much of the fear of the unknown, eases anxiety about controlling body reactions, and allows students to focus on methods of dealing with the symptoms. Knowledge is power to adolescents, and the more we can scientifically explain the operation of the voice or the body, the better our students will understand the physicality and complexities of singing. Perhaps they will also gain some respect for the human body along the way.

To return to the voice, I firmly believe that there are two main reasons why vocal anatomy and function are not discussed in many choral classrooms. The first is that many choral teachers simply do not understand basic vocal anatomy and function, so they do not teach it to their students. The second has largely to do with the fact that the larynx looks like a vagina, so much so that many music educators avoid showing pictures and diagrams in class altogether. As a profession, we have to completely disregard the appearance of the larynx and teach about it because that is part of our job as choral educators. In conference presentations, I often have attendees repeat after me, "The larynx is not a vagina!" People laugh loudly and awkwardly, but it is important that I acknowledge what most people in the room are thinking, especially when I start showing my presentation slides.

Following one of my lectures on female and male voice change at a state music conference, I spoke at length with two choral teachers at an evening reception. We talked and laughed about this issue. One of the teachers commented, "Why is it that photos of the larynx feel so personal? Would I feel the same about images of someone's liver?" Personally, I do not think so because I believe that we are socialized to think that private parts are private and best kept to ourselves (or only shared with whomever we deem worthy), but the visual similarity between the larynx and the vagina taps into deep cultural notions about what we have been taught to keep private. In fact, a beloved former University of Illinois colleague lovingly teased me whenever I shared the diagrams in presentations, saying, "Bridget, you are showing your porn again!" I always told him, "You know, you have one of these too." But his reaction was honest and is what I generally receive from people when I present images of the larynx.

After discussing the larynx during a conversation about vocal health in a summer graduate class, my Illinois graduate students gave me a laryngeal model at the conclusion of our semester together (see Figure 2.5).

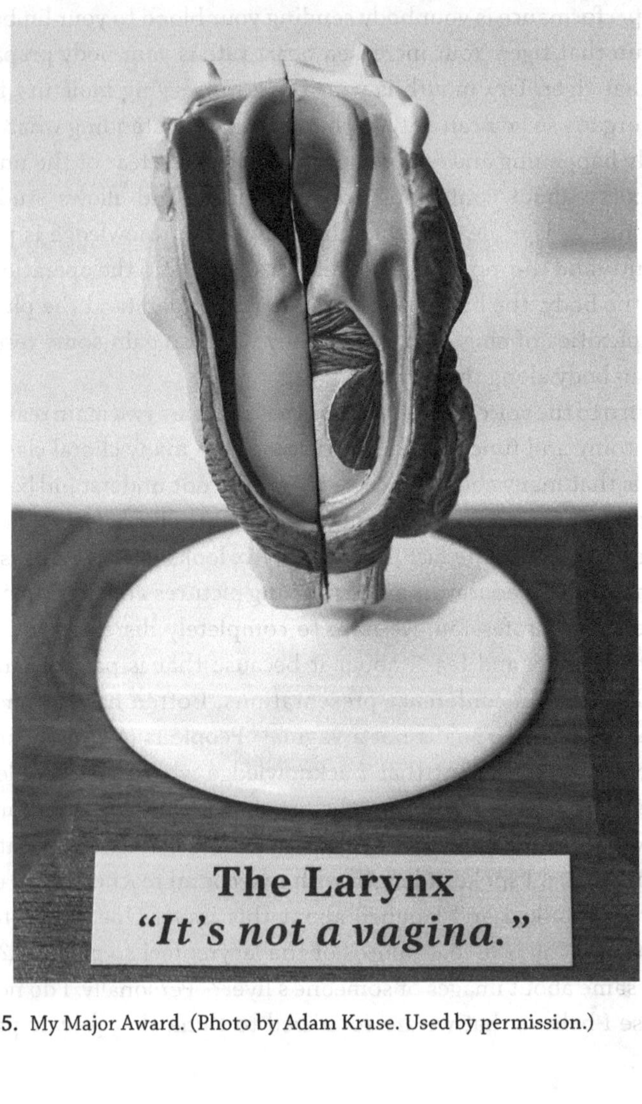

Figure 2.5. My Major Award. (Photo by Adam Kruse. Used by permission.)

My own personalized laryngeal model! I actually call this model-trophy my "Major Award" and do not know if I have ever laughed so much or felt so honored to receive anything before. If I go down in history associated with the phrase, "The larynx is not a vagina!" so be it. But I *do* know that people are listening, and I enjoy helping remove the stigma. The bottom line is that people need to get over how the larynx looks and teach about it because it is important and (almost) everyone has one.

I offer two disclaimers as we move forward: First, because adolescents process information differently, I advise discussing technical terms of anatomy and vocal function in conjunction with layman's terms and analogies or imagery. This works well alongside diagrams and models. Second, people of all ages can be squeamish. At one point two college students almost passed out in my Choral Methods class during the video portion of our discussion of laryngeal anatomy. It was the first time anyone has come close to passing out from footage in all the years of my presenting this discussion, but it was a good reminder that people can react in a number of ways to anatomical images. Be kind to your students (and yourself) if someone's instinct is to avert the eyes during visual portions of this conversation.

BASIC OPERATING PROCEDURES FOR THE LARYNX AND VOCAL FOLDS

The larynx is about the size of a walnut and sits in the neck just below the base of the tongue (see figure 2.6). An easy way to locate the larynx is to gently place a hand on the front of one's neck and say "Ahhhh!" It is located beneath the hand where you feel the vibration. The larynx is part of the respiratory system, which also involves the nostrils, tongue, soft palate, pharynx, trachea, lungs, and diaphragm. It has four main functions in humans: protecting the lungs from foreign material (food, liquid, vomit, and so forth); producing the voice; serving as part of the breathing tract; and helping stabilize pressure within the chest during activities such as lifting and straining (Heman-Ackah, Sataloff, & Hawkshaw, 2013). Nine separate cartilages are found in the larynx, as are many ligaments and tissue, and all are intricately connected and work together.

In 1741 Antoine Ferrien advanced understanding of the larynx in a presentation before the Parisian Academy of Sciences during which he used an excised dog larynx to demonstrate how the organ worked. Following his presentation (which was highly criticized, by the way) he wrote, "I approximated the lips of the glottis and blew strongly into the trachea; the

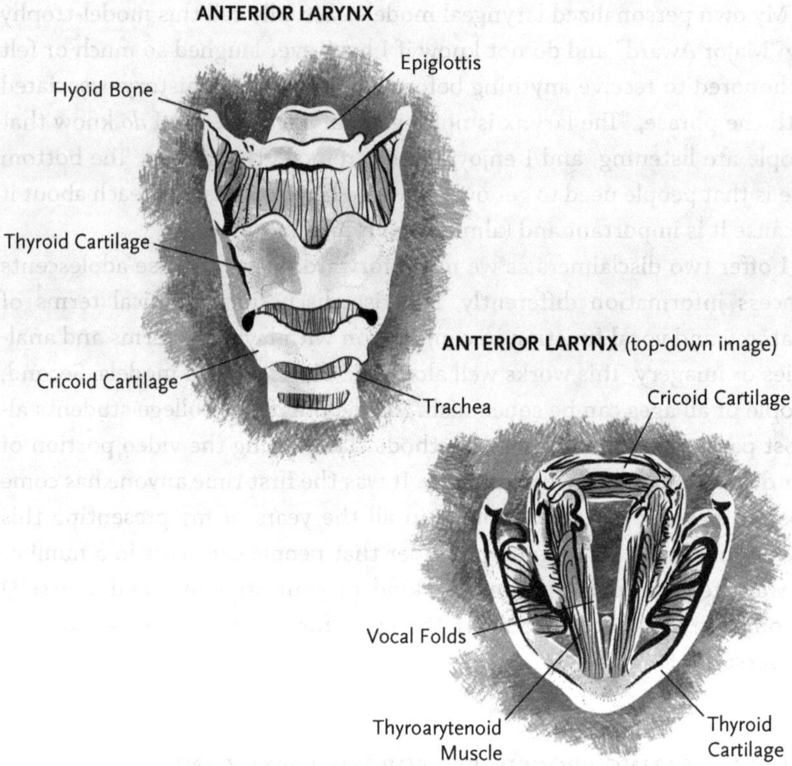

Figure 2.6. The larynx, anterior view. (Illustration by Kate Cosgrove, www.katecosgrove.com.)

organ seemed to become revitalized and produced not only a tone, but a real voice which was more pleasant to me than the most beautiful concert" (Luchsinger & Arnold, 1965, p. 69). Ferrien went on to coin the term *vocal cords* after comparing laryngeal anatomy with the strings of an Aeolian harp, which are also "set into vibration by an air flow" (ibid.).

Since Ferrien's time (and, yes, for more than 300 years) there has been great debate as to whether *vocal fold* or *vocal cord* is the proper term. The authors of the article "The Instrument of Voice: The 'True' Vocal Cord or Vocal Fold?" in the *Journal of Voice* (2017) considered the matter by examining historical vocal practice in using the terms. According to their research, the French physiologist Henri Detrochet (who discovered and named the phenomenon of osmosis) and the French experimental physiologist François Magendie (the first to prove the functional difference of the spinal nerves) countered Ferrien and recommended that the word *cords* be dropped in favor of *folds* because of "the observation that the vocal folds of the larynx did not act as a string instrument but acted more like the vibrating bands of wind instruments" (Hall, Cobb, Kapoor, Kuchai, & Sandhu, 2017, p. 133). The highly respected text *Gray's Anatomy: The Anatomical Basis of Clinical Practice* (Standring, 2016) acknowledged both terms but referred to this part of the larynx throughout the text as the *vocal fold*. *Gray's* conceded that *vocal fold* is the preferred clinical term though the terms can be used synonymously.

Many methods of laryngeal documentation have been used over the years, including still photography, cinematography, and videography, but initial documentation occurred in 1882. Thomas French of New York took the first successful photographs of the larynx in action in a live person (instead of a cadaver, as was standard practice until that point). He used a box camera with a laryngeal mirror attached, as well as a device to concentrate sunlight, and produced fairly high-quality black-and-white photos (Yanagisawa, Yanagisawa, & Sims, 2014, p. 303). Since that innovation in 1882, increased understanding about and visibility of the parts of the larynx have continued to fuel the debate about terminology. As the authors of "The Instrument of Voice: The 'True' Vocal Cord or Vocal Fold" point out:

> The development of laryngoscopy and microscopy has naturally led to far greater understanding of the mechanism of phonation itself and the microanatomy of the mucosal wave. As such, we contend that the term "fold" reflects best our modern anatomical and physiological understanding. To use the term "cord" etymologically suggests several strands, twisted, or woven together. Conceptually, the term "fold" neatly represents the pliability of the loose "outer" mucosal layers over the stiffer underlying vocal ligament and muscle. (Hall, Cobb, Kapoor, Kuchai, & Sandhu, 2017, p. 133).

At the conclusion of the paper the authors acknowledge that "language within medicine evolves in keeping with our understanding" and that *vocal fold* seems to be the best term moving forward. Therefore, I shall use the term *vocal fold* throughout this book.

In 1975 Minoru Hirano and his colleagues studied human laryngeal development and determined specific characteristics of vocal folds over the course of time. This groundbreaking research is still upheld today as the modern understanding of the microanatomy of the human vocal folds, and it was this work that determined the five different layers of vocal folds (see figure 2.7):

(1) The epithelium, which is of the squamous cell type. It can be regarded as a thin and stiff capsule whose purpose is to maintain the shape of the vocal fold;

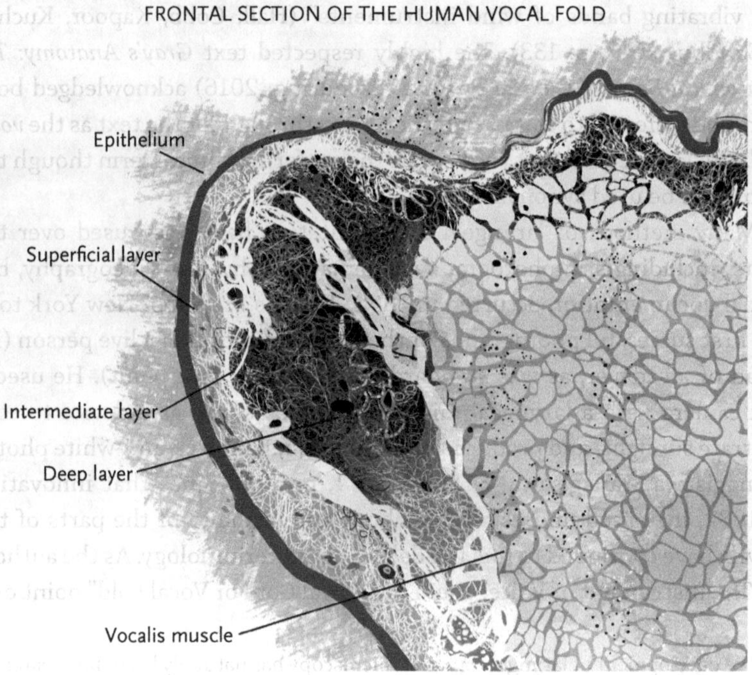

Figure 2.7. Frontal section of the human vocal fold. (Illustration by Kate Cosgrove, www.katecosgrove.com.)

(2) The superficial layer of the lamina propria, which consists of loose fibrous components and matrix. It can be regarded as somewhat like a mass of soft gelatin;

(3) The intermediate layer of the lamina propria, which consists chiefly of elastic fibers and can be likened to a bundle of soft rubber bands;

(4) The deep layer of the lamina propria, which primarily consists of collagenous fibers and resembles a bundle of cotton thread; and

(5) The vocalis muscle, which constitutes the main body of the vocal fold and is like a bundle of rather stiff rubber bands. (Hirano, 1981, p. 5)

Awareness of the intricacy and complexity of this organ is quite important. Does each cartilage, layer, or muscle need to be committed to memory? Absolutely not. But a solid understanding of and respect for this sophisticated instrument is essential, especially if you are a teacher working with developing singers who trust that you know what you are talking about.

When teaching adolescents about laryngeal anatomy and physiology, I want to foster an appreciation for the complexity of the organ, but most often start with basic descriptions so students can understand and appreciate what I am explaining without getting overwhelmed. Consider discussions about anatomy and physiology with your students as you would painting a room a dark color. Each conversation is another coat of paint on the walls. It takes time to build up the ultimately desired rich color, but each layer of paint will get you one step closer; each discussion builds on (and fills in some of the cracks of) the previous one.

My first conversation with adolescents about vocal anatomy usually begins with my saying, "If I were to cut off your head and look down your neck, this is what I would see" (it's good to have a nice attention-getting starter), and then I reference diagrams that show a top-down view of the larynx, vocal folds, and trachea such as figure 2.8.

When you consider this top-down view, it becomes very clear that vocal folds are positioned in the neck on the horizontal plane, not the vertical one. This is important for students to understand because (a) it reinforces the role of the trachea and breathing in singing, and (b) it prevents misunderstanding about how the vocal mechanism functions. Adolescent singers are notorious for straining their neck and head up or forward to sing a particular pitch; I call this technique "turtle necking." Since the vocal folds are in an anterior–posterior position in the neck (front to back) and parallel to the floor, external physical manipulation of the neck and head only creates more strain on the vocal mechanism and does not aid in reaching any particular notes. Understanding vocal anatomy and physiology can assist in

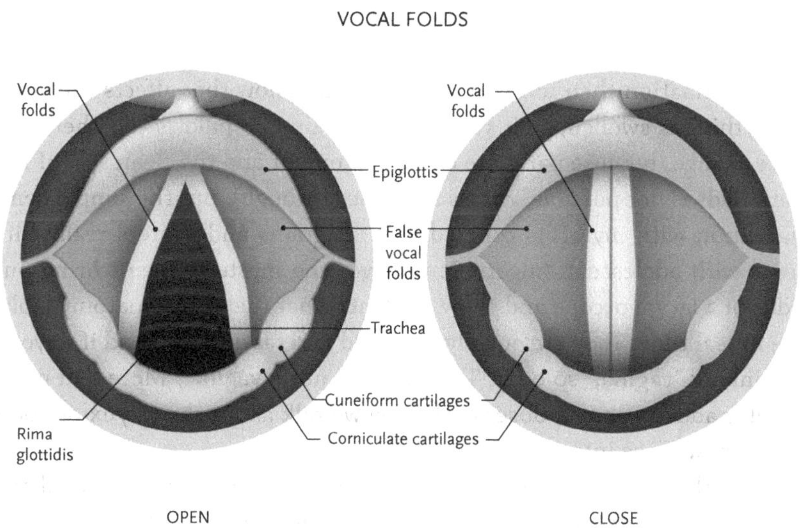

Figure 2.8. Vocal folds, looking down into the larynx and trachea. (www.Shutterstock.com [1098667472])

the prevention of potentially harmful or tension-inducing vocal habits in singers with changing voices.

After cutting off the imaginary head and orienting people to the top-down view diagram, I proceed along these lines:

> *(Holding my arms out in front of me, I close them together so that my forearms and hands are touching, from elbow to fingertips.)* My arms demonstrate your vocal folds, which zip and unzip like a Ziploc™ bag. When your vocal folds are zipped, air comes from the lungs below, pressure builds, and the air bursts through, causing your vocal folds to unzip and zip again very fast, creating the sound of your voice *(all the while making a fast "zipping" and "unzipping" motion with my forearms and hands).*
>
> Now, you may have heard of vocal nodes *(I have a volunteer make a fist with each of their hands and place their fists on the inside of my forearms, preventing my forearms from touching all the way)*, which are kind of like callouses on your vocal folds (and not how they describe it in the hit movie *Pitch Perfect*). Nodes come in pairs and polyps are singular; each affects how your voice works. There are many other voice disorders as well, but no discussion of those today. As you can see, because of the nodes on my vocal folds here *(student's fists on the inside of my forearms)*, I cannot zip my vocal folds cleanly across all the way. Not only can I not produce sound where those nodules are, there is extra open space between my folds now. What does that mean, then? *("Air comes through!" "Can't sing!")* Right! Excess air comes through the gap. And where the folds are not in contact, I cannot phonate there, which affects the function and sound of my voice.

The conversation then moves to laryngitis and how that affects the voice (everything is swollen, so it's like trying to zip two pillows together) and voice change (because parts are out of alignment and the clean seal of the vocal folds is not possible, excess air comes through). But the simple demonstration with my arms coupled with diagrams and posters really hits home with adolescent singers. It removes the mystery. *Then* I bring out video of a laryngoscope and show students what the actual anatomy looks like in real time. They are equally horrified and fascinated. (And if anyone is thinking "vagina," so be it. The larynx is not a vagina.) More and more detail is added in small doses each time we talk about the larynx or vocal function; we ease into it.

I like the user-friendly way in which Katharin Rundus described the phonation process in her book *Cantabile* in her quest to assist voice and choral teachers and students:

> The vocal folds are both loosely covered with a mucous membrane, which is an important factor in how they vibrate. The vibration begins when you deliver that slow, steady stream of well-coordinated air to your vocal folds. Voice scientists call this action myoelastic-aerodynamic. (Stay with me now!) Myoelastic means muscle (myo) that moves (elastic); aerodynamic means the motion of air and the forces that act on it. When air moves through your larynx on its way to your vocal tract, certain aerodynamic properties suck the vocal folds together and then re-open them in a physics principle called the Bernoulli Effect. As applied to singing, scientists call this action "flow phonation." At the same time, the "myoelastic" element works as a self-sustained oscillator, also contributing to a very complex vibration mechanism. Voice scientists refer to this complex vibration as "floppy," meaning that the muscle, ligament, and mucosa have the ability to vibrate in more than one mode, not just back and forth like sharply clapping your hands together, but like a ribbon undulating with many rippling motions. And remember that your vocal folds are very tiny; when they are closed (adducted), for men they are about 15–22 mm long; for women, 9–13 mm. What is really important for us to know is that this myoelastic-aerodynamic "floppy" vocal fold action, coupled with sharp, clean onsets, creates the most desirable complex vibration or sound wave. This is the raw material that is acted on in the resonators to create the most beautiful singing tone. (Did you get this far? Read it again if you need to. It is complicated but important.) (2009, p. 60)

Whereas movement of the vocal folds is generally easily understood, comprehending their actual length can be tricky. They are usually presented in a zoomed-in fashion in books and diagrams, making them appear much larger than they actually are. A typical wooden number two pencil is 7 mm in width, so female vocal folds (9–13 mm long) are a little bit longer than the width of a typical wooden pencil; the diameter of a dime is 17.9 mm, so male vocal folds (15–22 mm long) are approximately as long as a dime is wide. When the larynx and all of its parts are considered in true-to-life scale and shown via tangible example (i.e., a scale model, a student-created model, or lines of both lengths provided on a piece of paper), it is easier for adolescents to understand how a tiny shift (only millimeters!) in length *anywhere* in this walnut-sized organ throws off vocal coordination greatly in both females and males.

Conversations about vocal anatomy and function may take place during one class period or over the course of several, depending on the schedule. I do strongly believe that a big detailed discussion needs to take place with every choir at the start of *every* school year—regardless of who is new and who is returning to the choir. As adolescents mature and their voices change, they will each experience the lecture every year in a different developmental stage, and as stated above, will lock onto different information with each delivery. "Oh hey! I've had that problem recently!" "Yeeeahhh . . . that's happening to me now, too." I also enjoy including students in the conversations, having them share their own vocal experiences and talking about what is different now compared to last year. Such conversations remove stigmas concerning voice change, validate both female and male voice change experiences, and help foster a community that says, "Well, we are all in this together, so let's support each other through it. No laughing when funky vocal things happen because they are going to happen to almost everyone at some point." Providing a strong foundation at the start of each year additionally supports new students. As you reference and discuss the voice and voice change in different ways moving forward, everyone begins the choir year with the same solid understanding of vocal anatomy and function, as well as the same validation that they are normal.

OPERATING PROCEDURE DURING ADOLESCENT VOICE CHANGE

Adolescents benefit from understanding that voice change is, basically, just a growth spurt of the larynx. Voice change is not to be feared; it is the result of rapid and sporadic growth of a grouping of very small body parts. Adolescents have no control over the rate or amount of growth and development of their vocal mechanism, but knowledge about the developmental process reinforces the ideas that voice change will not last forever and what they are experiencing is different for everyone. Hang tight, because this too shall pass! Psychological and emotional facets of adolescent voice change are also worthy of discussion and will be addressed throughout the rest of the book.

Hormones initiate the process of voice change and ultimately determine harmonics of the voice for females and males:

> In the female, the impact of estrogens at puberty, in concert with progesterone, produces the characteristics of the female voice, with a fundamental frequency one third lower than that of a child. In the male, androgens released at puberty are responsible for the male vocal frequency, an octave lower than that of a child. (Abitbol, Abitbol, & Abitbol, 1999, p. 424)

As physiological growth progresses, the male larynx enlarges in a mostly front-to-back manner, whereas growth of the female larynx is more of a rounding in height and width (Abitbol & Abitbol, 2014; Abitbol, Abitbol, & Abitbol, 1999; Weiss, 1950). For males, "the thyroid cartilage enlarges significantly and the angle decreases to 90°, giving rise to the marked thyroid prominence known as the Adam's apple" (Mathieson, 2001, p. 102) (see figure 2.6). The term *Adam's apple* comes from the biblical story of Adam (the first man God created), who, according to the story, took a bite of a forbidden apple and a piece of it was forever stuck in his throat. The protuberance that we see in the male throat following puberty is (according to the biblical story) displaying the mark of Adam's sin.

A crucial detail of voice change is that everything in the larynx continues to move and function normally throughout vocal development; the organ does not operate differently than it always has. Issues arise because inconsistent and sporadic growth spurts in this walnut-sized organ result in many disruptions of alignment and coordination of the parts of the voice. Muscles of the larynx (for females and males) are weakened from sudden growth and thickening of the vocal folds, requiring "a constant reassertion of the muscle control skills needed for speech and singing" (Barlow & Howard, 2002, p. 67). Weakened laryngeal muscles cannot control the posterior (back) portion of cartilage of the larynx, which control the vocal folds, meaning that the folds remain somewhat open during phonation. Excess air permeates the voice through open spaces where the vocal folds do not make contact, resulting in a breathy or husky vocal sound that is characteristic of adolescent singers. Laryngeal gaps also create problems for the passagio, because the lack of closure prevents vibration from taking place, and from voice being produced, on the part of one fold that doesn't meet up with the other fold (Abitbol & Abitbol, 2014; Kahane, 1982; Luchsinger & Arnold, 1965).

Vocal folds, themselves, also undergo a growth spurt during voice change. For females, they grow 34% (approximately 3–4 mm) from prepuberty to puberty, resulting in a vocal range extension downward of about one third of an octave and upward of 3–4 pitches. For males, vocal folds grow 63% (approximately 1 cm) from prepuberty to puberty, resulting in a range extension downward of roughly one octave and up a sixth (Kahane, 1982; Luchsinger & Arnold, 1965). Three or four millimeters or one centimeter may not seem like much, but within an organ the size of a walnut, tiny amounts of growth can significantly impact vocal function.

Psychological and emotional components of voice change are as critical as physical considerations. Without encouragement from a trusted guide, and without an internal sense of drive and grit to persevere through vocal challenges, adolescents will not continue singing through voice change. In my book *Growing Musicians: Teaching Music in Middle School and Beyond*

(Sweet, 2016a) I wrote about the importance of helping adolescents persist in music classes during times of physiological upheaval and heightened self-consciousness, which seem to correlate with when they start making decisions about future involvement with music:

> At this peak time of great physical awkwardness and unpredictability, students start to make key choices about their musical involvement—largely based on current perceptions of their abilities at musical tasks. Again, *at a time when they are the most awkward*, students make big choices about their future involvement in music. It is a dangerous intersection for us as music teachers and we must proceed wisely to help our students feel successful and understand that physical skills will catch up to cognitive learning in due time, meanwhile keeping our music programs meaningful and relevant for adolescent musicians. (p. 7)

If students feel self-conscious and awkward and embarrassed while singing as a result of voice change, they will just stop singing. Why would they put themselves through painful physical or emotional experiences if they do not have to? Apart from physiological growth, psychological and emotional well-being play an enormous part in our work with adolescent singers and will be explored in chapter 3.

THE INFLUENCE OF HORMONES ON THE FEMALE VOICE

Although the intention of this book is to address both female and male adolescent voice change, this section of the chapter will specifically focus on female voices, for "voice problems related to sex hormones are encountered most commonly in female voice patients" (Sataloff, Emerich, & Hoover, 1997, p. 292). The human larynx has been identified as a "hormonal target organ" (Abitbol, et al., 1989, p. 157) and there is an abundance of information about hormones' influence on the voice in the field of voice science pertaining to birth, initial vocal development, puberty, the aging voice, pregnancy, transgender voice change, and more. I could write an entire other book on hormones and their influence on the voice. If you are interested in learning more than what I discuss here, the citations throughout this chapter and in the Additional Resources section are good starting places for further pursuing topics yourself.

In 1989 seven voice scientists published an article titled "Does a Hormonal Vocal Cord Cycle Exist in Women? Study of Vocal Premenstrual Syndrome in Voice Performers by Videostroboscopy-Glottography and Cytology on 38 Women" (Abitbol, et al., 1989) in which they compared uterine cervical cells with vocal fold cells. The researchers were unable to distinguish between the two samples and also observed basophil cells (a basophil is a basic white blood cell) in both samples. From this study, the scientists determined that there is, in fact, a menstruation-like cycle that takes place on the vocal fold epithelium (see figure 2.7). In addition, they determined that vocal folds are comprised of the same kinds of cells that make up our sex organs.

For this reason, the voice is exquisitely sensitive to any hormonal changes in the body, especially fluctuations of sex hormones (Kadakia, Carlson, & Sataloff, 2013; Vigil, 2015). As adolescent girls enter puberty, hormonal changes take place in preparation for the body's launch of menstruation that, in the process, affect vocal tissue and phonation. The collection of vocal symptoms that may result during pre-menstruation and menstruation is identified as premenstrual vocal syndrome (PMVS), also known as laryngopathia premenstrualis, premenstrual dysphonia, and dysphonia premenstrualis. In the chapter "The Larynx: A Hormonal Target" in the book *Diagnosis and Treatment of Voice Disorders*, 4th edition (2014) voice scientists Jean Abitbol and Patrick Abitbol kicked off their discussion of PMVS with a story:

> The premenstrual voice syndrome has been recognized for centuries. It has been reported by female singers at La Scala de Milano, at the Opera Houses of Vienna and of Salzburg, in the diaries kept by these opera houses. This suggests some explanation for the custom that used to be followed at European opera houses. For example, the female singers at the Opera of La Scala de Milano used to have "Grace Days." They were not asked to sing during the premenstrual period and while menstruating, but were still paid. Perhaps this abandoned practice should be reconsidered. (2014, p. 437)

So, what happens during PMVS? During premenstrual stages, concentrations of sex hormones in the body are drastically altered. Estrogen and progesterone levels decrease rapidly, preparing for menstruation. The dramatic shift in hormone levels contributes to vocal fold swelling, vocal fatigue, decrease in range, loss of vocal power, faint hoarseness, loss of range, and loss of agility. In addition, vocal folds respond to edema (swelling) by creating thickened mucus. All of this brings a temporary loss of suppleness of vocal fold tissue, resulting in disturbances in muscular and vibratory function. Plus, abdominal discomfort can lead to difficulties supporting vocal sound, emotional or mental blocks, and perhaps an increase in acid reflux. Abitbol and Abitbol (2014) also reported that body temperature changes influence laryngeal function. Before and after ovulation, body temperature increases; during menstruation, it drops. These changes influence laryngeal nerve response: when body temperature rises, there is an increase in the velocity of the conduction of nerve signals. When body temperature drops, there is a decrease in nerve conduction velocity (p. 438). Therefore, when adolescent females experience changes in body temperature related to hormonal changes, reaction times of the nerves in the larynx are affected.

In addition to physical readjustment and re-coordination of the larynx and all the parts within it, adolescent singers—especially females—also experience vocal challenges on a cellular level as a result of hormonal flux. Although PMVS has been documented for centuries, there is a PMVS-shaped void in choral music education. The more I dig into the voice science literature, the more I find, and the more curious I am about why this topic is not addressed more adamantly. My biggest hunch is that conversations about hormones and menstrual cycles feel much too personal for choral teachers, especially with adolescent students. Kimberly Mullendore Brown addressed this in her article "Sex Hormones and the Female Voice: Communication in the Voice Studio":

> Our society, more often than not, views the topic of menstruation as an uncomfortable, awkward, and private matter. Consequently, the subject is often taboo in the voice studio, preventing open communication about a student's menstrual cycle symptoms, even if both student and pedagogue understand the importance of such communication. (2015, p. 447)

I get the awkwardness, I really do. And I certainly do not advocate beginning rehearsal with, "So, ladies, let's talk about your menstrual cycles." But keep in mind that the research discussed here was conducted with adult women with regulated hormonal cycles. As teachers of adolescent students in the throes of puberty who are experiencing hormonal fluctuations on an hourly, daily, and weekly basis, we should not turn a blind eye to this very real aspect of female voice change. In her article "Premenstrual Syndrome and Its Effects on Laryngeal Functionality: An Approach for Singers and Pedagogues," Erin Oberlander wrote, "While discussing women's health issues may seem awkward or indiscreet, if a student is in fact a sufferer of PMVS, a voice teacher's refusal to help deal with the situation is pedagogically unsound" (2010, p. 32).

My University of Illinois colleague and friend, Professor Yvonne Redman, was for 18 years a main-stage soprano at the Metropolitan Opera in New York. In addition to performing and teaching voice, she is also becoming a noted scholar of vocal pedagogy and health. She's also one of my favorite people with whom to talk about all things related to the larynx (it's good to have one of those). From Yvonne, I have learned that the influence of hormones on the voice is often discussed in the field of vocal performance, especially with regard to vocal health. In her own voice studio, Yvonne discusses hormones with her female collegiate voice students. She notes:

> With new students I do not approach the subject until a comfortable rapport has been established—this time varies depending on the student's personality—but usually a few weeks into the semester after we've covered repertoire selection, IPA, and diction. I discuss it casually under the unofficial heading, "Vocal fatigue, recognizing its symptoms and factors that contribute to it." I usually start with lack of sleep, dehydration, vocal overuse and acid reflux. I then explain how our monthly cycles can affect us and the tissues we use to sing; this is most often the case during the premenstrual stage (PMS). I also discuss how this stage can worsen all of these symptoms. The best we can do is be aware of "heaviness" in our instrument and body and adjust our behaviors to counteract these warnings of fatigue. I then beat into their brains the importance of staying away from anything except Tylenol™ when they feel swelling in their vocal folds. Tylenol™ does not weaken blood vessels, which is why hospitals use it. All other painkillers weaken vessel walls and can lead to hemorrhage. Because females tend to have ectasias on their vocal folds during hormonal changes, the vessels get closer to the surface with swelling; you do not want impact to rupture the vessels. [Ectasias are enlargement or dilation of capillaries on the surface of the vocal folds. Some believe this to be an estrogen effect similar to "spider veins" that one might see on the legs.] If my students experience vocal fatigue in any form longer than a couple of weeks it's time for a doctor's visit. So far this has served the students (and me) well. One student discovered she has ectasias close to the surface of her folds, and this is a very important conversation to have with someone like that. With all students I find that mentioning the words "menstruation" and "period" are very unpleasant and stay away from them completely by using "PMS" and "monthly cycle." (Yvonne Redman, email communication, shared with her permission)

I greatly respect Yvonne and the important work she does both within and outside her studio. Her insight is important to the conversation about adolescent voice change and the broader music community, especially with regard to broaching the topic of PMVS with sincere intentions backed by refereed research and motivated by a desire to empower female singers.

As music educators, we need to know as much as we can about possible contributors to vocal challenges for singers whose voices are changing. It is also important and possible to talk to our adolescent singers (especially females) about the influence of hormones on their voices so that they better understand why their voices work or feel differently from day to day. In conversations about vocal anatomy and physiology, we can easily include remarks such as, "As your bodies are working their way through puberty, you will all experience hormone fluctuations which can affect how your voice functions and feels from day to day. Come see me if you are concerned about a change in your voice or about how it feels when you sing." Framing the influence of hormones in such a way bypasses all mention of menstruation or PMVS and provides information and encourages awareness among your adolescent singers. What is most important is to encourage self-advocacy of such singers, to get them to recognize what "normal" vocal function generally feels like for them, and to inform them that the hormones in their body will affect their voices in addition to laryngeal growth and re-coordination.

Permit me to end this section with a quick story: In one of our conversations, Yvonne shared an interesting fact from the not-so-distant past. Some European opera houses allowed main-stage female singers to wear a red rose or flower on their dresses to signify that they were mid-menstrual cycle and, therefore, audience members and critics should be kinder when listening to them sing because their voices may not be in top form as a result. Fantastic!

DIGEST

An understanding of vocal anatomy and physiology can empower both female and male adolescent singers as well as the teachers assisting them through the voice change process. Access to information helps ease adolescent fears of vocal challenges and validates the voice as a complex and impressive instrument worthy of deeper appreciation. It is imperative that reference to vocal anatomy and physiology be ongoing so that students gain a solid foundation of knowledge from repeated exposure to ideas, but also so that they may continually "re-place" themselves in the scenario over time as their own instrument matures. In addition to comprehending the physiological aspects of voice change, adolescents should also be instructed in the importance of monitoring their own instrument, advocating for their voice, and maintaining an open dialogue with their teacher during vocal challenges and development.

Also, the larynx is not a vagina.

CHAPTER 3
Strength from Within

Courage doesn't always roar. Sometimes courage is the quiet voice at the end of the day saying, "I will try again tomorrow."

Mary Ann Radmacher

And I know it's hard when you're falling down
And it's a long way up when you hit the ground
Get up now, get up, get up now

Imagine Dragons, *On Top of the World*

Throughout life, everyone encounters challenges and obstacles, successes and accomplishments, failures and defeats. To counteract negative happenings in my life, I employ mantras or personal theme songs and anthems to motivate me through what comes my way. Songs, poems, images, and symbols that represent or demonstrate resilience are especially appealing to me. For example, one of my favorite choral texts is the hymn "How Can I Keep from Singing?" It is attributed to the American Baptist minister Robert Wadsworth Lowry:

> My life flows on in endless song;
> Above earth's lamentations,
> I hear the real, tho' far-off hymn
> That hails a new creation;
> Through all the tumult and the strife
> I hear its music ringing;
> It sounds an echo in my soul—

How can I keep from singing?
Although the tempest loudly roars,
I hear the truth, it liveth.
But though the darkness 'round me close,
Songs in the night it giveth.
No storm can shake my inmost calm
While to that rock I'm clinging;
Since love is lord of heaven and earth,
How can I keep from singing?

When tyrants tremble, sick with fear,
And hear their death-knell ringing,
When friends rejoice both far and near,
How can I keep from singing?
In prison cell and dungeon vile,
Our thoughts to them are winging;
When friends by shame are undefiled,
How can I keep from singing?

This text is mighty and moving, and I enjoy singing these words as, yes, they stir my soul. I also enjoy exploring this text and others akin to it with adolescent singers, who eagerly tap into messages of determination and riding out tough times. When working with people—whether it be in a college course, a middle school choral festival, a high school workshop, or a teacher in-service—I make it a priority to reinforce ideas of strength, perseverance, and self-care in various forms as a takeaway from our time together. The longer I am an educator, the more I am aware of the increase in anxiety, tension, stress, self-criticism, perfectionism, and depression in the world around me, and no age group or profession seems exempt. A little kindness and empathy can go a very long way.

When considering adolescent voice change, all stakeholders may find themselves experiencing stress, doubt, fear, and anxiety during the process. This goes for the adolescent singer as well as for their teacher. It is okay to say out loud that voice change can be difficult—*really difficult*—for all involved, but it is good to maintain perspective. It is not most difficult for *us*, the teachers; it is most difficult for our students. We might experience moments of frustration while teaching the changing voice, but they pale in comparison to what some adolescents are experiencing at this stage. Our work as music educators compels us not to be distracted by personal frustrations stemming from students' vocal limitations, which are completely out of their control, but to empower our students to navigate vocal challenges during physical upheaval. Our students will definitely benefit if we can demonstrate an *onward ho!* spirit about the whole experience.

During times of great vocal challenge, if the psychological and emotional needs of adolescent singers, female and male, are not met, it is likely that they will not work through vocal difficulties and will stop singing. Until coordination of the vocal mechanism returns, students must be provided with *something* to keep them going, to keep them from quitting. This chapter focuses on ideas of resolve that are essential to the navigation of voice change. These ideas mainly involve our being adolescent singers' biggest advocates and cheerleaders. So get ready! For this chapter, you are going to need your pom-poms.

> *And I know it's hard when you're falling down*
> *And it's a long way up when you hit the ground*
> *Get up now, get up, get up now.*

GRIT, VULNERABILITY, AND RELENTLESSNESS

Perspective is a powerful idea, especially in the context of adolescence. Although adolescents are intelligent and often insightful, I have generally found them to struggle with keeping the bigger picture in mind, whether that be the bigger picture of friendships, physical development, academic achievement, social perspective, concept of happiness, or something else. When discussing adolescents with my University of Illinois music education students, I demonstrate adolescent perspective by putting one hand close to the front of my face to represent where adolescent focus typically remains and stretch the other hand far away from my face, representing the idea of the bigger picture. It is challenging to see the bigger picture—the outstretched hand—with the closer hand consuming most of my field of vision. Adolescents often perceive their world similarly as they (using the hand analogy) largely maintain focus on what is immediately in front of them and struggle to see the bigger picture or anything in the distance. Our work with adolescents can increase their abilities to perceive more of the bigger picture, to better see what is possible rather than only what is immediately in front, but it takes time.

As discussed in the first two chapters, adolescents have little control over many aspects of their physical development. This lack of control contributes to physical awkwardness and can lead to a rise in self-consciousness, confusion about self-concept, and a lowering of self-esteem. These responses, in turn, may contribute to feelings of inadequacy, especially with regard to musical ability. As mentioned earlier, it is often during this time of intense, sporadic, awkward physical development and intense emotion that adolescents reach a crossroads about continuing participation in music. If they are not feeling good about their voices as a result of voice change challenges, they may elect to stop singing altogether when provided the opportunity.

Perseverance is one of the most important components of successful navigation of voice change for adolescents, but unfortunately, it is not addressed often enough in choral music. Again, if adolescent singers do not feel good about themselves, they will quit singing. But if they feel positive about their efforts and are acknowledged for doing many things well—as well as they can in the moment—there is a greater chance that they will stay with singing long enough to see the physiological pieces coordinate again and continue singing with increased confidence and ability.

I understand that talking about perseverance with adolescents does not guarantee that they will continue to sing throughout middle and high school or that they will be music educators or life-long singers. There are many reasons why people sing and many reasons why they do not. If singing is not for a particular student, no problem, and I wish that student all the best in discovering their own interests and passions. But what I can barely stand is the thought that adolescents leave singing because of shame or embarrassment about their voice. I want students to know that their voices will continue to develop and grow well into the second and third decades of their lives, that voice change is only *a drop in the bucket* of all possible voice experiences to come. If an adolescent decides not to sing, I hope that it is with a full heart and understanding about the voice and simply because they want to try something else, not because of frustration or misunderstanding of the big vocal picture.

Just as conversations about anatomy and physiology are woven into the fabric of music rehearsals and classroom culture, so should concepts of perseverance. The larger idea of perseverance is known by varied names including resolution, stick-to-it-iveness, resilience, determination, drive, persistence, and tenacity. What follows is a brief look at the idea of perseverance under the designations of grit, vulnerability, and relentlessness. I encourage you to consider each of these with regard to your own music classroom and ruminate on how you might embed these concepts in your teaching practice in order to empower and encourage your adolescent singers through voice change and vocal challenges.

Grit

Angela Duckworth is the author of the *New York Times* bestselling book *Grit: The Power of Passion and Perseverance* (2016), in which she unpacks the ideas of personal potential and drive, as well as talent. Ultimately, her message is that you do not have to be the smartest or best at something to be highly successful at it. What matters is not talent or intelligence but perseverance through the challenges and obstacles; that's what she means by *grit*. Success comes from the grit or grittiness within you that pushes you and drives you to continue and not give up. After reading *Grit*, I consider myself a really gritty person. During my career, there have certainly been times when I have not been the strongest musician in the room or the person who knows the most about a topic. But I know deep down that I have a voice to share and a perspective that is valuable, so I will put myself out there almost every time. I do not shy away from a challenge, even if it terrifies me. I am creative about finding solutions to problems and do not throw in the towel at the first, second, or third hiccup. I recognize that I am gritty.

Duckworth's book has been highly praised and highly criticized, and I have found both the book and the criticisms to be fascinating (look at both sides of the conversation; some starting places are provided in the Additional Resources section at the back of this book). For the purposes of the current discussion of adolescent voice change, I think the idea of grit translates extremely well into our work with singers with changing voices. No matter how well you sing or how well you can control your vocal mechanism before or during voice change, what gets you through it is your willingness to push through the challenges and obstacles as your body grows and realigns. The more grit you have, the more likely you are going to keep singing during voice change and make it to the other side (and have some fun along the way).

Voice change affects adolescents' ability to sing, right? Some adolescents have an easier time with vocal challenges during voice change, allowing them to demonstrate more vocal ability than others. Because voice change can last for a significant period of time, it is a short walk from perceptions about a student's ability (meaning literal control of the voice) to perceptions about the student's talent (meaning whether or not they have a special musical skill). It is important that teachers working with changing voices understand that the stages of adolescent ability development are long and often full of ups and downs, and students should never be considered on the basis of "talent." Here are Duckworth's thoughts about talent:

> Is talent a bad thing? Are we all equally talented? No and no. The ability to quickly climb the learning curve of any skill is obviously a very good thing, and, like it or not, some of us are better at it than others. So why, then, is it such a bad thing to favor "naturals" over "strivers"? What's the downside of television shows like *America's Got Talent, The X Factor*, and *Child Genius*? Why shouldn't we separate children as young as seven or eight into two groups: those few children who are "gifted and talented" and the many, many more who aren't? What harm is there, really, in a talent show being named a "talent show"? In my view, the biggest reason a preoccupation with talent can be harmful is simple: By shining our spotlight on talent, we risk leaving everything else in the shadows. We inadvertently send the message that these other factors—including grit—don't matter as much as they really do. (2016, p. 31)

Duckworth's theory of grit has two parts. The first part is: talent × effort = skill. The second is: skill × effort = achievement. She writes,

> What this theory says is that when you consider individuals in identical circumstances, what each achieves depends on just two things, talent and effort. Talent—how fast we improve in skill—absolutely matters. But effort factors into the calculations *twice*, not once. Effort builds skill. At the very same time, effort makes skill *productive*. (2016, p. 42, emphasis in original)

With singers undergoing voice change we have to consider this formula a little differently because, first of all, circumstances are *never* identical during this process. Puberty influences physical development differently in every person. Second, ongoing physiological growth of the larynx and learning to re-coordinate all the parts is a unique process and takes a different length of time for each person. Therefore, I fully support throwing the term *talented* out the window with regard to adolescents. The really important part of this formula in connection with voice change is that effort builds skill and then more effort makes skill productive. This part of the formula is quasi-magical when we consider persevering through voice change: working hard and making progress will ultimately result in good things, regardless of what happens along the way. As Walt Disney said, "Around here, however, we don't look backwards for very long. We keep moving forward, opening up new doors and doing new things, because we're curious . . . and curiosity keeps leading us down new paths" (McKim & Anderson, 2007).

Instead of focusing on student talent during voice change, what if we maintained focus on grit? Yes, aim for musicality and singing in tune *as much as possible* (side note: I sincerely love the buckshot pitch-matching sound that is so characteristic of changing voices), but treat clawing forward and upholding emotional expression, effort, and attitude as what matters most as the voice resettles and blossoms. How might students react? How might middle-level choral and voice teachers react? How might high school and collegiate choral teachers benefit? I think this shift in focus within choral education would motivate adolescents to use their voices more overtly, be more willing to take risks and sing in front of each other, and actually accomplish more in the long run. I imagine that choral teachers who work with changing voices would also feel less pressure about results. They would have more space to focus on individual adolescent voices and to maintain awareness of where singers are *today*. Teachers would also have more time and opportunity to celebrate all small and large moments of progress as beautiful and worthy of a fuss.

When I taught middle school choir at Kenneth T. Beagle Middle School, I was always proud of my students when they sang in performances, as they had worked *so* hard. The problem was that no one else really knew how much we had bled and sweat to sing this well in tune; how much we had labored to be there. Unfortunately, some festival adjudicators did not have their ears calibrated for middle-level singers and were unable to consider all we had accomplished behind the scenes to sing as well as we had. Today, I keep notions of grit and forward progress at the forefront, making sure that my singers understand the messages and emotions of their songs, revel in the harmonies of their pieces, feel empowered by sharing their voices, and have fun. When I adjudicate at festivals, I do my best to provide helpful feedback for their future work as singers while honoring and recognizing what they have clearly been working on to sing for me today.

Reimagining Duckworth's formulas for our work with changing voices might look something like this:

Original Grit formula, part 1: talent × effort = skill

Voice change modification: ~~talent~~ changing voice [present ability] × effort [a huge aspect, because this is what can actually be controlled] = skill at the moment [some increase in skill level, dependent on present ability]

Original Grit formula, part 2: skill × effort = achievement

Voice change modification: skill at the moment [present ability] × effort [a huge aspect, because this is what can actually be controlled] = celebrated achievement [any accomplishment, no matter how big or small; there is a wide spectrum of possibilities]

There are some aspects of adolescent voice change that singers and choral educators can control, and many that they cannot. Understanding the difference is important and encouraging the most appropriate aspects, such as effort, is key. Celebrating all accomplishments, both great and tiny, may encourage adolescents to dig further into their grit storage and keep persevering. I also recommend that we, the choral educators, continue to tap into our own supplies of grit, especially in times of frustration or exasperation, so that we can model perseverance and continued effort for our adolescent singers.

Vulnerability

Brené Brown is a research professor at the University of Houston well known for her studies of vulnerability, courage, authenticity, and shame. Her book *Daring Greatly: How the Courage to Be Vulnerable Transforms the Way We Live, Love, Parent, and Lead* (2012), was a *New York Times* bestseller and more than one million copies have been sold since publication. Much of her discussion can be applied to our work with adolescent changing voices. We want adolescents to walk into our "choral arena" with courage and willingness to engage in singing, daring greatly to share what only they can share, and engaging with symptoms of voice change with courage. She writes:

> Vulnerability is not weakness, and the uncertainty, risk, and emotional exposure we face every day are not optional. Our only choice is a question of engagement. Our willingness to own and engage with our vulnerability determines the depth of our courage and the clarity of our purpose; the level to which we protect ourselves from being vulnerable is a measure of our fear and disconnection.
>
> When we spend our lives waiting until we're perfect or bulletproof before we walk into the arena, we ultimately sacrifice relationships and opportunities that may not be recoverable, we squander our precious time, and we turn our backs on our gifts, those unique contributions that only we can make.
>
> *Perfect* and *bulletproof* are seductive, but they don't exist in the human experience. We must walk into the arena, whatever it may be—a new relationship, an important meeting, our creative process, or a difficult family conversation—with

> courage and the willingness to engage. Rather than sitting on the sidelines and hurling judgment and advice, **we must dare to show up and let ourselves be seen.** This is vulnerability. This is *daring greatly*. (Brown, 2012, p. 2, emphasis in original)

Brown's book is so full of ideas that are applicable to working with adolescents that it is a little overwhelming to parse out what to share here. With acknowledgment that there is much more that could be explored, I will keep to her ideas from chapter 2, "Debunking the Vulnerability Myths."

Myth #1: Vulnerability Is Weakness. Brown argues that vulnerability is not a good or a bad thing; it's just a thing.

> It's not what we call a dark emotion, nor is it always a light, positive experience. Vulnerability is the core of all emotions and feelings. To feel is to be vulnerable. To believe vulnerability is weakness is to believe that feeling is weakness. (p. 33)

If vulnerability is perceived as weakness, and feelings or emotions are also considered weakness, then our work as choral music educators is doomed. However, if we promote the idea that emotions are important, that the way students feel is not wrong, and that being vulnerable to feelings allows them to experience singing on greater and deeper levels, we can foster new ways for students to interact with music, as well as life in general.

Brown goes on to say that "vulnerability sounds like truth and feels like courage. Truth and courage aren't always comfortable, but they're never weakness" (p. 37). One of the ideas that I promote with my Illinois music education students is the importance of establishing the classroom as a safe space for adolescents to be themselves to explore new facets of their identity as people and as musicians. Safe spaces are not *sterile* spaces, however, and feeling safe is not the same as feeling comfortable all the time. As adolescents explore who they are and navigate vocal changes, there will be moments of tension or joy or sadness or anger or frustration or exhilaration, and so forth. What is felt in a certain moment is not right or wrong; it is how a person feels at that moment. For adolescents, feelings and emotions ebb and flow a lot, and it is important to acknowledge that these feelings are not *wrong*. We can provide spaces where adolescents are free to feel vulnerable and further unpack and decipher how they are feeling and thinking. With more awareness of their emotions, singers may be able to experience choral music—and voice change—in more meaningful and empowering ways.

Myth #2: I Don't Do Vulnerability. Although people would like to avoid feeling this way, vulnerability permeates our daily lives whether we like it or not. And as Brown says, "Unfortunately, there is no 'get out of vulnerability free' card" (p. 43). Adolescents who are navigating voice change feel exposed and vulnerable when they sing because they never really know what sounds are going to come out of their mouths. These feelings of vulnerability can promote negative emotions of fear, self-doubt, and anxiety, which perpetuate Myth #1, that vulnerability is weakness. As we know, many adolescents will stop singing altogether to avoid such emotions, so how can we infuse power back into their experiences of vulnerability? Brown writes,

> When we pretend that we can avoid vulnerability we engage in behaviors that are often inconsistent with who we want to be. Experiencing vulnerability isn't a choice—the only choice we have is how we're going to respond when we are confronted with uncertainty, risk, and emotional exposure. (p. 45)

We can empower adolescents during voice change by promoting the idea of choice. They may not have the power to perfectly control their voices, but they have the power to choose their response to their vocal adversity (with the caveat that this idea would work best if students already understood the anatomy and physiology of their changing voices). When something wonky happens with the voice, adolescents have the power to *choose* whether they will dismiss it as normal and "how it is at the moment," they can *choose* to be upset by it, or they can *choose* not to engage in singing activities at all. Students cannot avoid feeling vulnerable, but they certainly are not powerless. We need to make sure that they understand that.

Myth #3: Vulnerability Is Letting It All Hang Out. In order for adolescents to engage fully in singing, they must feel connections to the music; without personal connection, they will lose interest and may not continue to sing. *Personal connection* means that students have tapped into a memory, experience, relationship, emotion from their own lives and aligned it with the text or meaning of the music they are learning (or learning about). Class activities or discussions intended for fashioning personal connections with music may lead adolescents to feel vulnerable because they are recalling emotionally charged personal information. Sometimes this recall is best done silently with oneself; other times it is best accomplished within a full group of students. Let the circumstances and class dynamics be your guide.

While feeling vulnerable is an important part of the process of connecting with music, it does not mean that our students (or we teachers) have to share *all* our personal details:

> Vulnerability is based on mutuality and requires boundaries and trust. It's not oversharing, it's not purging, it's not indiscriminate disclosure, and it's not celebrity-style social media information dumps. Vulnerability is about sharing our feelings and our experiences with people who have earned the right to hear them. Being vulnerable and open is mutual and an integral part of the trust-building process. (p. 45)

What matters most is that students trust us as their teachers and know that their personal experiences will be honored within the conversation and in the classroom, whether they wish to share their experiences aloud or not.

Myth #4: We Can Go It Alone. The following chapters of this book delve into emotions associated with adolescent voice change, including feelings of isolation and sadness. Whereas voice change is complex on a physical level, it is also complex on an emotional level. It truly is an experience rooted in vulnerability, if ever there was one. After quoting Whitesnake's "Here I Go Again," Brown dispels Myth #4, that vulnerability is best traversed alone:

> Well, as much as I love the idea of walking alone down a lonely street of dreams, the vulnerability journey is *not* the kind of journey we can make alone. We need support. We need folks who will let us try on new ways of being without judging us. We need a hand to pull us up off the ground when we get kicked down in the arena (and if we live a courageous life, that will happen). (p. 53, emphasis in original)

More than anything, our students need to feel supported by us, their teachers. They need our encouragement, support, and lack of judgment throughout their challenges. Again, voice change is not easy and vulnerability plays a big part, but if choral teachers and adolescent singers approach it with the right mindframe, the experience can be empowering, enlightening, and restorative for all involved. So I'll see Brown's Whitesnake and raise her a Foo Fighter; the chorus to their song "Times Like These" could be an anthem for our adolescent singers:

> It's times like these you learn to live again.
> It's times like these you give and give again.
> It's times like these you learn to love again.
> It's times like these time and time again. (Grohl, Hawkins, Mendel, & Shiflett, 2003)

Relentlessness

Personal development expert Gary John Bishop published *Unfu*k Yourself: Get out of Your Head and into Your Life* in 2017; it quickly made the *New York Times* bestseller list. His book is organized into chapters titled as personal affirmations: I am willing. I am wired to win. I got this. I embrace the uncertainty. I am not my thoughts; I am what I do. I am relentless. I expect nothing and accept everything.

Part of the chapter "I am relentless" applies to this discussion of the adolescent changing voice. Consider the following passage with regard to adolescent singers (who want to be involved in singing) and their teachers (some of whom want to work with such students, and some of whom do not); also keep the notion of the invisible audience in the back of your mind.

> Anytime you're working to achieve something, you're going against the current. Often the opinions of the people around you are trying to push and pull you away from your destination.
>
> They'll say you can't do it, you're making a mistake, it's impossible, you'll fail. The more unique and out-of-the-box your endeavor is, the stronger the push-back can be. Why? Well, mostly because the other people in your life have gotten used to relating to you as a specific "kind" of person. So anytime you attempt to break out of that mold, you're not only messing with your own world, you're also messing with theirs.
>
> And the resistance doesn't just come from other people; it comes from your own mind too. Both your conscious and unconscious thoughts can work against you to stop your dreams right in their tracks.
>
> And when you inevitably stumble or encounter some sort of obstacle, you question the journey at all. Maybe it's even time to turn back.
>
> At this point, when you don't know whether you're up or down, how far you have to go or how far you've come, there's only one thing that can keep you going.
>
> That thing is relentlessness. The momentum to keep moving and moving and moving, no matter what happens. (pp. 145–146)

Bishop's idea of relentlessness aligns with concepts put forth by Duckworth (*Grit*) and Brown (*Daring Greatly*), but it was Bishop's emphasis on battling resistance outside yourself in combination with resistance from within that struck a short, concise chord with me regarding adolescent voice change.

In chapter 1 of this book, "The Adolescent," I discussed how scrutiny was constantly present in the lives of our adolescent students. Much of what Bishop outlined in his chapter reminded me of the external scrutiny applied to changing voice singers by forces such as mass media and music educators who disdain working with this population. External scrutiny also comes from the invisible audience—always watching, always trying to push or pull adolescents in different directions, stressing failure, influencing the ways our students speak to themselves. Internal resistance could include feelings of anxiety about singing, fear of embarrassment and vocal unpredictability, frustration at not being able to control the voice, and so forth. Regardless of the source of the pressures or resistance that adolescents may feel about singing or their changing voices, our work as choral educators calls us to empower singers and help them tap into the relentlessness within to keep moving forward, no matter what.

This passage also speaks to choral educators, especially those who genuinely enjoy working with middle-level singers but feel pressures from friends, family, or the larger profession to strive for something else. Experiencing external resistance against something that we want to do or believe in is frightening and powerful. It will either sway us to change or more firmly root us in what we want and where we are. Internal resistance could include self-doubt and feelings of inadequacy that manifest in imposter syndrome. In my career, I have experienced external resistance from people about my wanting to be a middle school educator and then again about my wanting to teach college. I have fought internal resistance that caused me to wonder if I have made the right choices or if I am making a difference. Ultimately, I have to keep believing in what I do and what I want to do, and recognize that relentlessness is an important and ongoing part of my empowering myself to accomplish my goals.

DIGEST: PERSEVERANCE IN PRACTICE

As mentioned at the start of this chapter, the idea of perseverance should be woven into the fabric of the classroom and referenced on a regular basis, alongside the anatomy and physiology of the voice. One-and-done discussions about grit and resiliency are not going to be meaningful and are not going to stick; the idea of relentlessness should be a well-known facet of your choral program. For example, when I taught choir at Kenneth T. Beagle Middle School, I hung a poster that said "Make an effort, not an excuse" over the chalkboard in the front of the classroom. When students whined about having to stand while singing because it was [any day of the week], I would not say anything but would point at the sign. When students sang something in a lazy fashion and blamed it on [fill in any season or weather condition], I would point at the sign. But when students sang with gusto and effort, I would say something along the lines of, "That was wonderful! We have things to work on, yes, *but* you sang with so much effort! No matter what, you did not stop! I am really proud of you. *Great effort.*" In my classroom, students knew that effort was one of the things that mattered most: not perfect pitches, not perfect voices, not perfect complexion, not perfect clothes, not perfect behavior. If you showed up and made an effort, it was going to be a great experience. And in the long run, effort promotes energy, which results in singing more in tune, with more expression, better articulation, and so forth. When students put forth effort, it all evened out nicely in most cases.

The same holds true with the adolescent choirs I work with today. At some point during our time together, I tell them,

> I am not looking for a technically perfect performance in the concert because I can hear one of those any time I want. I can forgive wrong notes or rhythms, as long as you are doing your best to sing as accurately as you can. But the one thing that *must* happen during the performance, no matter what, is that you bring yourself into the music and show the audience that you know what you are singing about and have somehow connected with each song. I can hear a technically perfect performance any day, but I do not hear a performance that *moves me* very often. You have the capability to move every single person who hears you sing at the concert. *That is our goal.* Put your effort into compelling your audience into believing what you are performing *and* enjoy yourself. Then it will be amazing, no matter what happens otherwise.

And my singers get it. They understand what I am saying because they know what is compelling and interesting and what is lazy and minimal effort. They are not stupid and they will do the least they can get away with, just like most human beings on the planet. But then they go out on the stage and *get it,* meaning that they sing their hearts out and they move people's emotions. I give them permission to let go of fear of perfection and be gritty, resilient, and relentless in all the moments. They understand that if they make a mistake, it is okay as long as they are making an effort; they know that I am not going to be mad at them if something unforeseen happens while they are trying. What matters is that they persevere and continue making music, singing, and expressing themselves—that they do the best that they can.

Some forms of perseverance that I promote with students (and practice myself) include the following:

- *Mantras.* A mantra is a phrase or slogan repeated frequently. Mantras can help in a specific moment or have a cumulative effect when repeated over time. They could benefit adolescent singers when used as a strategy to counteract frustration from voice cracking and so forth. It could be something along the lines of, "I am safe. I am important. I am normal. I am healthy." They can also be helpful when read repeatedly, so perhaps they could decorate your office or classroom. Here are a few of my favorite mantras:

  - Act your way into a new way of thinking.
  - You've got this.
  - Eat the elephant one bite at a time.
  - One foot in front of the other.
  - Do the best that you can with the time that you have.
  - You do you.
  - Be yourself.
  - What lies behind you and what lies in front of you pales in comparison to what lies inside of you. —*Ralph Waldo Emerson*
  - The devil whispered in my ear, "You're not strong enough to withstand the storm." Today I whispered in the devil's ear, "I am the storm."
  - I can and I will.
  - I can and I am.
  - Only when we're brave enough to explore the darkness will we discover the infinite power of our light.—*Brené Brown*

- *Theme songs or personal anthems.* In moments when we do not feel strong or we feel overwhelmed, it is nice to have a theme song or personal anthem to hum, sing, or listen to as a way to change our spirits or empower us. There are days when I get out of bed and start singing my theme song in my head immediately so that I keep moving forward toward the day; it helps put pep in my step right away. Some days I listen to my theme song 10 to 15 times in a row to calm me or get me through a challenging task. My anthems pump me up when I am excited or nervous; I feel like I'm surfing on sound. Sometimes my theme songs are a warm hug when I cannot do anything about my circumstances but feel sad feelings. As a musician, I gain a great deal from personal anthems and can customize them according to what I need, cognitively and emotionally. This is a concept that adolescents understand well—listening to music to navigate and validate emotions—and we can tap into that to help them persevere through times of challenge and struggle with their changing voices or whatever else comes their way.
- *Self-reflection.* Although self-reflection can certainly involve journal writing, there are many ways to be reflective including video journaling, painting, haiku, songwriting, beat making, blogging, meditation,

dancing, and filmmaking. We can guide adolescents with changing voices through activities of self-reflection pertaining to topics of personal wellness, singing ability, vocal challenges, successes and frustrations, methods of perseverance, and concepts of the future self. The possibilities for self-reflection truly are countless, and the benefits are even more abundant.

Hey! I'm not giving up today!
There's nothing getting in my way.
And if you knock, knock me over
I will get back up again!
Oh! If something goes a little wrong,
Well you can go ahead and bring it on.
'Cause if you knock knock me over, I will get back up again!

"Get Back up Again" from *Trolls* (Mitchell & Dohrn, 2016)

CHAPTER 4

Voice Change in Pop Culture

Pop culture and entertainment can be dismissed as surface, but it's not. It's the language we all speak, and it's the connection point between people all over the world.

Bozoma Saint John

In all the years I have worked with adolescent singers, in all the readings I have encountered, and in all the forms of media I have watched, I cannot recall expressions of enjoyment about experiencing voice change. I am not talking about choral teachers who enjoy working with adolescent singers but about the actual experience of voice change. Because it can be an extremely challenging aspect of puberty for females and males, I am not surprised.

Complicating matters, I have frequently read about the practice of dismissing young boys from choirs after their voices showed signs of change. They were dismissed because their voices had (and I quote) *broken*. This practice has spanned centuries and is alive and well today, but the notion that changing voices could be considered something broken breaks my heart. I am immediately reminded of the scene in *Toy Story 2* (Plotkin, Jackson, & Lasseter, 1999) in which the cowboy doll, Woody, has a nightmare about his broken arm. In this scene Woody is asleep and dreaming about his owner, Andy, who excitedly grabs him to play. Suddenly Andy remembers that Woody is broken and falls into a zombie-like trance, saying in an emotionless monotone, "Oh. I forgot. You're broken. I don't want to play with you anymore." Andy then glazes over, extends his arm, and drops Woody into a bottomless garbage can where he falls and falls into an abyss. Woody wakes up, screaming.

I can only imagine the devastation experienced by the many boys who loved singing and were then suddenly dismissed. Adding insult to injury is the fact that the entire voice change experience is out of the control of the singer, which would make being considered broken that much more painful. The choral director Frederick Swanson was an ally of the young male singer and was very vocal about his opposition to the idea of a changing voice as something broken. In his 1973 book *Music Teaching in the Junior High and Middle School*, he wrote:

> The voice "break" came to be a dreaded event, a dismissal and a deprivation of opportunity for schooling. . . . There was nothing to be done about it; no reputable vocal coach or musical director would take a youth as a student at this time. It never occurred to anyone that this might be a subject for study or research, and that it might be possible to salvage all of those fine years of training and keep this "veteran" in an activity for which he was so well prepared. No, it was simply one of those things about which nobody could do anything. "His voice is a poor broken thing. His period of usefulness is at an end. He must be dismissed." (Swanson, 1973, pp. 180–181)

In addition, misunderstandings have perpetuated stigmas about changing voices for centuries. One example comes from the article "Voice Change in Human Biological Development" by emeritus professor of history Herbert Moller, who described the beliefs of Johann F. Oest (1787), whom he quotes:

> Toward the end of the eighteenth century, when many boys experienced an earlier mutation of their voices than their elders considered normal, anxious educators found a deep voice in a teenager disturbing. A German educator was convinced that early voice change was a sure sign of masturbation: "In cities, where choirs exist, one should especially watch out for boys who sing soprano parts. If their treble voice darkens before they are seventeen, even though they observe the dietetic rules of a soprano singer, it is obvious what is the matter with them." (Moller, 1985, p. 241)

Another example of misunderstanding comes from the 1800s, when many renowned singers and medical professionals believed that a broken voice was akin to a broken bone in the body (more on that in chapter 5). Further, well into the 20th century it was believed by many respected people that if a boy had any hopes of singing as an adult, he should refrain from all singing throughout the entirety of his voice change. Singing during this transition was thought to be one of the worst things a person could do for their voice.

Fast forward decades to a time when information is mainly distributed via a popular culture that has evolved to include music, television, movies, apps, games on smartphones, and more. Whereas mainstream understandings about voice change were spread by word of mouth and publications by revered individuals in centuries past, today they are in large part perpetuated by portrayals in mainstream media. This chapter aims to provide insight into the role that pop culture can have on today's understandings and perceptions of the adolescent changing voice.

SIMULACRUM

In his 2016 article "Featherless Dinosaurs and the Hip-Hop Simulacrum: Reconsidering Hip-Hop's Appropriateness for the Music Classroom," my music education colleague at the University of Illinois, Adam Kruse, used the term *simulacrum* to describe the general reaction of music educators to the idea of using hip-hop in the music classroom. He couched his argument in a brief discussion of the movie *Jurassic World* (Trevorrow, 2015), in which dinosaurs appear as featherless creatures. This portrayal of dinosaurs goes against recent research claiming that dinosaurs actually may have had feathers and fur. Kruse explained that movies such as *Jurassic World* do not have dinosaurs with these features because the general population believes dinosaurs to look like, well, what you typically would think a dinosaur looks like: no fur or feathers. So the movie reinforces the societal belief or assumption that dinosaurs do not have fur or feathers, which then becomes a situated reality that is not based in fact but accepted in pop culture. Kruse wrote about this with regard to his agenda of promoting the use of hip-hop in school music programs and the way a simulacrum has complicated that effort:

> This type of simulated reality is what philosophers have called a simulacrum. While a complete exploration of the concept is beyond the scope of this article, I employ here the notion forwarded by the French philosopher, sociologist, and theorist Jean Baudrillard that a simulacrum can become its own form of reality. This means that the simulacrum of featherless dinosaurs found in mediated representations has generated its own reality and movies like *Jurassic World* exist within that reality. A simulacrum also exists relating to hip-hop music. This simulacrum states that hip-hop music is saturated by and promotes violence, drug use, misogyny, materialism, and a litany of other antisocial values and behaviors. Based on this simulacrum, many music educators might feel that hip-hop is inappropriate for inclusion in the classroom. (Kruse, 2016, p. 14)

I can also apply the idea of a simulacrum to adolescent voice change, for the generally embraced perception of the experience is that it is one of humiliation, anxiety, turmoil, and dread. While voice change is not always pleasant, people perceive and approach the experience with such angst and trepidation well before it begins that it is rarely given the opportunity to be something positive or exciting. In *Simulacra and Simulation*, Baudrillard states:

> It is no longer a question of imitation, nor duplication, nor even parody. It is a question of substituting the signs of the real for the real, that is to say of an operation of deterring every real process via its operational double, a programmatic, metastable, perfectly descriptive machine that offers all the signs of the real and short-circuits all its vicissitudes. Never again will the real have the chance to produce itself—such is the vital function of the model in a system of death, or rather of anticipated resurrection, that no longer even gives the event of death a chance. (Baudrillard, 1994, p. 2)

I agree that much of what is generally "known" about adolescent voice change is rooted in a substitution of attitudes about the real for the real, itself. I acknowledge that there are many choral music educators who enjoy working with adolescents through their voice change (and I am one of them), but there are many more who dismiss adolescents solely on the basis of misunderstanding or negative perception of the changing voice. If this weren't the case, I would not have bothered writing this book.

There is a bit of "wagging the dog" with all of this as well, which means that something of lesser importance in a situation takes on the role of prime importance. Media portrayals of voice change tend to focus on the unpredictable, the humiliating, the negative, and this then becomes what people know and expect of the experience of voice change. Although the challenges do exist, there is much more to the experience of voice change than just negativity, fear, and brokenness. Positive aspects include the fact that voice change means development of the adult voice, with which a person can sing and speak in many new ways; that understanding of what is happening physiologically during voice change can make it easier to navigate the challenges; that a sense of pride and accomplishment comes from gaining access to new notes and colors to the voice; that a sense of community or peer mentoring can be fostered among adolescent singers as they all go through this together, female and male; and that students can learn to laugh at the experience and not take themselves too seriously. Although shades of the positives are included in pop culture portrayals, negative facets receive the primary focus, perpetuating a simulacrum of voice change. As Baudrillard asks:

> Are the mass media on the side of power in the manipulation of the masses, or are they on the side of the masses in the liquidation of meaning, in the violence perpetuated on meaning, and in fascination? Is it the media that induce fascination in the masses, or is it the masses who direct the media into the spectacle? (1994, p. 84)

What follows are transcriptions and detailed descriptions of three popular television shows from three different decades that featured well-known storylines of male adolescent voice change: *The Brady Bunch*, *The Wonder Years*, and *The Goldbergs*. After the three transcripts, I consider what is portrayed and reinforced about voice change experiences and puberty, especially over time. For ease of following each episode, I formatted the transcripts as screenplays.

The Brady Bunch

The Brady Bunch first aired in 1969 and ran until 1974. It was the story of a lovely lady named Carol, who was bringing up three very lovely girls, Marcia, Jan, and Cindy. All of them had hair of gold, like their mother; the youngest one in curls. It's also a story of a man named Mike Brady, who was busy with three boys of his own, Greg, Peter, and Bobby. They were four men living all together, yet they were all alone—until the one day when the lady met this fellow, and they knew it was much more than a hunch that this group must somehow form a family. That's the way they all became the Brady Bunch. And along the way they were joined by their live-in housekeeper, Alice.

In 1972 the *Brady Bunch* episode "Dough Re Mi" (season 3, episode 16) revolved around Peter's voice change (he was the middle son of the blended family). At the beginning of this episode, Peter answers the phone and is mistaken for one of his sisters.

<begin transcript>

Peter answers the ringing telephone; his voice is high and squeaky; we only hear one side of the conversation.

PETER

Hello? Oh, hello Sam! Marcia?! *I'm not Marcia!* No, I'm not Jane either! (squeaky) I'm *Peter*! She's barbecuing right now. Okay, I'll tell her. Bye!

Peter heads outside to where Alice is grilling hamburgers.

PETER (to ALICE)

Alice, that was Sam. He said he'd call back later. He thought I was a *girl*!

<end transcript>

Meanwhile, the oldest brother, Greg, has written a song called "We Can Make the World a Whole Lot Brighter," which he is positive is a "sure-fire hit song . . . a gold record!" Greg wants to record the song in the "best recording studio in town" and convinces his brothers and sisters to form a singing group called The Brady Six; they pool their allowances to help pay the studio rental fees. The recording session is booked for Friday afternoon and all is ready to go! That is, until . . .

<begin transcript>

All six siblings are in the family room, singing through "We Can Make the World a Whole Lot Brighter." Mrs. Brady and Alice are in the kitchen putting dishes away; they can clearly hear the rehearsal taking place in the next room. The scene jumps back and forth between the family room and kitchen.

THE BRADY SIX

(*singing*) . . . *Let's go out and try to make it better.*
And maybe we can make the world a whole lot (*Peter's voice suddenly cracks*) *brighter,*
We can make the load a little lighter.

(in the kitchen) MRS. BRADY

Uh-oh. Somebody sure hit a clinker.

THE BRADY SIX

(*Peter's voice cracks and creaks repeatedly as the group sings together*) *Everybody has to try together . . .*

GREG

(*frustrated*) Alright, Pete. Quit the clowning.

PETER

(*confused*) Who's clowning?!

(in the kitchen) MRS. BRADY

Augh! That was worse than a clinker.

(in the kitchen) ALICE

That was a *clunker*!

GREG

Alright, let's try it again from the top of the bridge. One, two three . . .

THE BRADY SIX

(*singing*) *And maybe we can make the world a whole lot* (*Peter's voice suddenly cracks*) *brighter,* (*Peter's voice keeps cracking and squeaking*) *We can make the load a little* (*big crack*) *lighter.*

GREG

(*irritated*) What's the problem?!

PETER

(*confused*) I'm not doing it on purpose, honest!

(in the kitchen) MRS. BRADY

(*with a concerned look on her face*) Alice, how old was Greg when his voice started to change?

(in the kitchen) ALICE

Around thirteen, I think . . . (*a look of sudden realization crosses her face*)

(in the kitchen) MRS. BRADY

Uh-oh.

(in the kitchen) ALICE

Maybe you're right. When Sam called the other day he said that Peter sounded like a girl. I bet Pete's voice was cracking then.

Greg and Peter enter the kitchen and open the refrigerator for a pitcher of water.

GREG

Maybe some water will get rid of that frog.

PETER

My voice is sure doing *goofy* things lately.

MRS. BRADY

Hey, the group was beginning to sound really good in there!

ALICE

Yeah, right on!

PETER

(*voice squeaking with a big high crack*) Thanks! (*He immediately looks at Greg, confused.*) A lot.

MRS. BRADY

Peter, I don't know how to tell you this, but I'm afraid your voice is . . . *changing*.

PETER

(*squawking*) My voice?! (*looking confused, puts his hand to his throat*) *Changing?*

GREG

(*a horrified look crosses his face*) OH, NO. We're supposed to record Friday! That's only six days away!

PETER

How long does it take a voice to change?

MRS. BRADY

(*gently*) Well . . . it's . . . hard to say.

GREG

(*very upset*) We gotta record my song *Friday*! I gave Mr. Dimsdale $150 *nonreturnable* dollars!

PETER

Don't worry, Greg! By Friday my voice is gonna be just (*huge crack*) *swell*!

SCENE CHANGE: In Peter and Greg's shared bedroom, Peter is sitting with his head over a humidifier, tented with a towel. When he lifts his head, large amounts of steam roll out.

GREG

How you doin', Pete?

PETER

(*from under his towel tent*) I think I'm starting to melt!

GREG

Cheer up! The steam is beginning to help. Your voice sounds like it used to!

PETER

Yeah! I think it's (*loud crack of his voice*) back!

GREG

Here . . . (*Greg pulls out a jar of honey and a spoon*) take some of this honey. Here it comes! (*Greg puts honey on a spoon and sends the spoon up under the towel to where he assumes Pete's mouth is located.*)

PETER

(*from under the towel*) Not in my ear!

GREG

Sorry.

PETER

Hey that tastes pretty good!

GREG

(*excited*) Say that again! I think the honey is working already!!

PETER

I said, that tastes pretty (*voice cracks loudly*) good!

GREG

Stand by for more honey . . .

PETER

Are you sure honey is good for the voice?

GREG

Sure! You've never heard a bee's voice crack, did ya? (*Peter pulls back the towel and looks at Greg.*)

<end transcript>

Later that evening, Mrs. Brady wakes up in the middle of the night to a loud wailing sound that seems to be coming from downstairs. She wakes Mr. Brady and the two of them quietly sneak downstairs to see what's happening. They literally run into Alice, who is investigating the same strange noise. Mister Brady thinks it might be a coyote, and Alice suspects it is a mountain lion. Their search leads them to the driveway, where they find Peter lying in the front seat of the family car trying to "scream [his] voice back to the way it was." Alice goes back to bed, and the parents climb in the car with Peter to have a talk.

<begin transcript>

PETER

(*frustrated*) Of all the crummy times for my voice to change!

MRS. BRADY

Oh, honey. It's all part of growing up! (*snickering*) You should have heard my brother when his voice changed! He sounded just like my mother! (*laughing*)

MR. BRADY

(*laughing*) Yeah, you should have heard me when I was your age! (*speaking in a very high voice with occasional squeaks throughout*) Good morning, mother! Good morning, father! (*laughing*)

PETER

(*still frustrated*) Why couldn't my voice start changing (*squeaking*) after Friday? By then we could have recorded Greg's song and everybody wouldn't look at me *that way.*

MR. BRADY

There are some things that you *just have* to leave to Mother Nature. It will pass.

PETER

(*bitterly*) I hope Mother Nature has to record a song someday and her voice starts to crack.

MR. BRADY

Maybe your voice won't crack on Friday.

PETER

(*sadly*) I sure hope it doesn't because I don't want to let the others down.

<end transcript>

Two days before the big studio recording session, the rest of the Brady Six (minus Peter) votes on whether to keep Peter in the group for Friday's recording session or tell him he can't join them. They are all very torn about what to do, with two of them voting to keep Peter and two voting to kick him out. Cindy, the youngest, is undecided. Their mother walks through the room while the conversation about Peter is taking place, and the kids ask her what she thinks they should do.

<begin transcript>

```
                    MRS. BRADY
Look kids, listen, I could make the decision for
you, but it wouldn't be right. I would like to
give you something to think about, though. You
know, money and fame are very important things,
but sometimes there are other things that are more
important . . . like, people.
```

<end transcript>

The siblings decide to call off the recording session just as Peter graciously bows out of the group in order not to create any problems with his cracking voice. The siblings feel really bad for Peter but don't know what to do. Off-handedly Greg says, "We can't record with Peter's voice changing all through the song. Or can we?" and then he runs off and writes a new song called "Time to Change." Not only is the song about growing up, Mother Nature, and voice change, but it incorporates Peter's cracking voice as an actual part of the song. Here are the lyrics:

Sha na na na, na na na na na, sha na na na na
Sha na na na, na na na na na, sha na na na na

Autumn turns to winter, and winter turns to spring.
It doesn't go just for seasons, you know, it goes for everything.
The same is true for voices, when boys begin to grow.
You gotta take a lesson from Mother Nature, and if you do you'll know.

Chorus:
When it's time to change, then it's time to change.
Don't fight the tide, come along for the ride, don't you see?
When it's time to change, you've got to rearrange
who you are into what you're gonna be.

Sha na na na, na na na na na, sha na na na na
Sha na na na, na na na na na, sha na na na na
Day by day, it's hard to see the changes you've been through.

A little bit of living, a little bit of growing all adds up to you.
Every boy's a man inside, a girl's a woman too.
And if you wanna reach your destiny, here's what you've got to do!

Chorus × 2

The episode "Dough Re Mi" ends with a little outro that reveals that the Brady Six decided that Peter's cracking voice is now going to be their singing group's trademark sound; plans have been made to record more songs in the studio *featuring* Peter.

The Wonder Years

The Wonder Years was a popular television series that ran from January 1988 to May 1993. Kevin Arnold (actor Fred Savage) was the main character, and the show revolved around his experiences from early adolescence into adulthood during the 1960s and 1970s. Other main characters included his parents, his older brother and older sister, his best friend Paul Pfeiffer (actor Josh Saviano), and the love of his life, Winnie Cooper (Danica McKellar)—although through most of the show, Winnie had little idea about the extent of Kevin's affinity for her. The show also featured the voice of The Narrator (Daniel Stern), who was supposed to be Kevin as an adult, reflecting on the happenings of his youth.

In my opinion, one of the greatest episodes of *The Wonder Years* was the one titled "The Glee Club" (season 3, episode 16), which first aired on February 27, 1990. I appreciate this episode even more today as a teacher of adolescent singers and a teacher of music teachers than I did at the time, when I watched it as an adolescent with a major crush on Fred Savage.

<begin transcript>

RFK JUNIOR HIGH SCHOOL

As the camera pans down various school hallways, snippets of different choral songs are heard, sung beautifully in different languages by different choirs.

NARRATOR

The halls of RFK Junior High often echoed with the sounds of music. The Kennedy Chorale. The Kennedy

Madrigals. And of course, the Kennedy Now-Tones. They were all part of a long-standing family of song. But, as with every family, there was a skeleton in the closet.

Camera pans into a music room with a male teacher sitting behind the piano facing a large group of adolescent boys who are singing arpeggios on an "ah" very, very loudly and harshly and out of tune.

NARRATOR

The boys' eighth-grade Glee Club. The singing group from hell.

The teacher, Mr. Frace, looks distressed and says "Oh boy" at the singing in a disappointed tone.

NARRATOR

Twice a week we transformed Mr. Frace's choir room into a kind of chamber of musical horrors.

Mr. Frace says "Oh my gosh" as the camera focuses on individual male students' faces as the loud, harsh, out-of-tune "ahs" continue.

NARRATOR

Randy Mitchell, baritone.
Doug Porter, monotone.
Paul Pfiffer, no tone at all.
And of course . . . *me.* Not that we didn't have heart. It's just that the 13-year old male voice isn't exactly designed for . . . well . . . for *singing*.

Mr. Frace stands up at the piano saying, "Hold that note," and the boys hold individual pitches on "ah!" No one is matching the pitch of the people around him. While the boys hold the note very loudly and largely out of tune, Mr. Frace walks to a window in the choir room that looks into the math classroom next door. Clearly the loud, unpleasant sound is leaking into that room, as a female math teacher is glaring back at Mr. Frace in a disapproving manner.

NARRATOR

We weren't the stuff that Tabernacle choirs were made of. So out of respect for the arts, and humanity, we reached the agreement: we wouldn't push Mr. Frace if he wouldn't push us.

Mr. Frace turns around and half-yells to the loud group of boys holding their individual "ah" tones.

MR. FRACE

ALL RIGHT!! That's enough!! Just get out your books and study.

The room turns silent as the boys sit down on the choral risers and get out their books and papers.

NARRATOR

All in all, a pretty equitable arrangement.

PAUL (to KEVIN)

It isn't fair! Every other group gets to sing some songs and stuff! Why can't we?

KEVIN (to PAUL)

Well, maybe because we *stink.*

PAUL (to KEVIN)

Well, then *why* are we here?

FELLOW EIGHTH GRADE BOY

Because we *have* to be here. Right, Warren?

He turns to a tall, dark-haired, good-looking young man reading a book in the back row of the choir risers, Warren Gander. Warren doesn't move his head away from his book, but his eyes move and look back at the boy speaking to him, expressionless.

NARRATOR

Warren Gander. No one had ever heard him sing a note. Much less say a word.

PAUL (to KEVIN)

So what you're saying is we're *losers*. Is that it?

All of the boys look at each other and nod a small nod, indicating "yes."

NARRATOR

But if Paul was looking to unite us in chorus . . .

All of the boys in the room suddenly turn to Paul and blow out a long raspberry at him.

NARRATOR

. . . he had just heard our best effort. Face it. We knew where we stood. At the bottom of the heap. And we were smart enough to not seek the limelight.
Until . . . that is . . .

It's a new school day and the boys are walking into the choir room, talking quietly in small groups and taking their places on the risers. The blinds are suddenly raised and sunlight pours into the room. The boys are shocked and look quickly toward the blinding window. There stands Ms. Haycock, a petite woman in her early 20s, dressed in a blue skirt suit with hair in a stylish hairdo of the times, with a giant, perky smile on her face.

NARRATOR

. . . the limelight was thrust upon us.

MS. HAYCOCK

There! That's better, isn't it?

Ms. Haycock bounce-steps to the piano, hands in excited fists by her side as all the boys look at each other in great confusion.

KEVIN (to PAUL)

Who's she?

Ms. Haycock sits at the piano and plays one big chord.

MS. HAYCOCK

(*chant-singing the words all on one pitch*) *My name is Ms. Haycock.*

The camera pans to the shocked boys, one of whom is holding a pencil in his teeth, which falls out of his mouth when his jaw drops open in surprise.

MS. HAYCOCK

(*chant-singing*) *And if there is anything I want to impress upon you, it's . . .*

Plays another loud chord up one step from before.

MS. HAYCOCK

(*still chant-singing*) *. . . Use your diaphragms! Always use your diaphragms!*

Ms. Haycock places her hand near her ribs to indicate where the diaphragm is located. The boys look at her and each other with confused and horrified looks on their faces.

FELLOW EIGHTH-GRADE BOY (to KEVIN)

What'd she say?!

Ms. Haycock, smiling broadly, plays a third chord on the piano, moving up one whole step from the last. She continues in a full, cheerful voice.

MS. HAYCOCK

(*chant-singing*) *Do you hear how that sounds? Full and supported?*

Ms. Haycock plays a fourth chord, again moving up a melodic step and chant-singing in the new key. The boys continue to look horrified.

MS. HAYCOCK

(*chant-singing*) *If you're doing it right, you'll feel it down here!*

Ms. Haycock perkily gestures toward her lower abdomen, and the camera focuses on a confused-looking eighth-grade boy, seated on the risers, who immediately looks down at his lower abdomen in horror and swallows his gum in a giant gulp-swallow. Ms. Haycock plays another loud chord on the piano and continues to chant-sing in the coordinating key.

MS. HAYCOCK

(*chant-singing*) *I'm thrilled to be taking over the eighth-grade boys' Glee Club!*

Ms. Haycock plays a chord and moves up a key.

MS. HAYCOCK

(*chant-singing*) *And when we sing, we'll always sing like this!*

Ms. Haycock plays another chord and the boys look at each other with expressions of amusement and disbelief on their faces.

MS. HAYCOCK

(*chant-singing*) *Because we're always going to remember to use our . . .*

Ms. Haycock finishes her chant-singing introduction in the original key where she began on the piano. She freezes in place, with a hand behind her right ear, broad smile on her face, looking at the boys, and waiting for them to finish her sentence. A long silence. No one moves.

ALL MEMBERS OF THE EIGHTH-GRADE BOYS GLEE CLUB

(*a quiet, awkward mix of mumbling, speaking, and feeble singing*) Diaphragms.

Ms. Haycock smiles and gives a little nod at the boys.

NARRATOR

She was fresh out of teaching school. Full of ideas. And, oh yes! The woman was a total lunatic.

IN THE BOYS' LOCKER ROOM

PAUL (to KEVIN)

Well, I think she's great.

KEVIN (to PAUL)

Paul, get a grip.

PAUL (to KEVIN)

Why? Just because she sang a little?

KEVIN (to PAUL)

A *little*?! I just hope she doesn't think we're gonna sing like that.

PAUL (to KEVIN)

Well, maybe not at first. But once we master this diaphragm thing . . .

Kevin gives Paul a look that says, "Don't be so sure."

NARRATOR

Diaphragms or no diaphragms, Ms. Haycock's arrival had sent a shudder of fear through all of us.

EIGHTH-GRADE BOY 1 (to KEVIN and PAUL)

I don't *want* to sing. That's why I took Glee Club in the first place.

<end transcript>

The boys continue talking among themselves about Ms. Haycock and her work as a student teacher. The boys collectively decide that Ms. Haycock needs to put on a good front as the student teacher but will soon tire of them and Glee Club will go back to the way it was before with Mr. Frace. That, however, is not what happens. Instead, Ms. Haycock launches voice auditions, during which several of the boys are featured singing a portion of the song "America."

<begin transcript>

IN THE CHOIR ROOM, EIGHTH-GRADE BOYS' GLEE CLUB REHEARSAL

NARRATOR

It was time to show Ms. Haycock exactly what she was up against. In other words, it was time to sing.

PAUL

(*singing loudly, boldly, largely out of tune*) *My country, 'tis of thee . . .*

EIGHTH-GRADE BOY 1

(*singing loudly, higher in range, a raspy voice that breaks and squeaks constantly*) *Sweet land of liberty . . .*

EIGHTH-GRADE BOY 2

(*singing loudly, almost entirely on one pitch*) *Of thee I sing!*

EIGHTH-GRADE BOY 3

(*singing loudly, on the same pitch, but in a different key from the piano*) *Land where our fathers died . . .*

WARREN GANDER

(*He stands silent and stoic, staring off into the distance, and doesn't open his mouth or make a sound.*)

KEVIN

(Loudly, overly dramatic, almost entirely in tune, many arm moves) From every mountain side, let freedom ringggg!

<end transcript>

Shortly afterward, Ms. Haycock presents the boys with music for the song "Stout-Hearted Men." The response is one of shock and horror, as the Narrator exclaims, "No one but no one had ever threatened us with an actual musical arrangement!" The teacher goes on to announce that the choir will be performing "Stout-Hearted Men" at the Spring Sing Concert in a month. The boys react with a shocked "What?!" and the Narrator shares the boys' inner monologue, "And suddenly it was clear. Our reputation was on the line here! Our tradition. Our bad name." Kevin tries to tell Ms. Haycock that the boys are not interested in learning the song or performing, but his conscience gets the best of him. Instead, he implies that everyone is fine with it, much to the dismay of his classmates.

Over the following weeks, Ms. Haycock teaches "Stout-Hearted Men" while cheerfully praising them ("Splendid!") and reminding them, "Diaphragms! Diaphragms!" The boys are not singing well in every sense of the word; they are singing out of tune, singing too loudly, and not singing together at the same time. In short, it is a mess. Their teacher seems oblivious to the sounds that the boys are actually producing and her demeanor is never less than one of joy and positive perkiness. In the meantime, Kevin is being taunted by his friends for not revealing their true feelings about singing at the Spring Sing: "You got us into this, you gotta get us out. Our lives are depending on it."

<begin transcript>

Back in the choir room, eighth-grade boys' glee club rehearsal

Ms. Haycock is seated behind the piano, playing the bass line for "Stout-Hearted Men" with her left hand and conducting a nonstop two pattern with her right hand. She is looking at the boys with a huge, unwavering grin and proclaiming sentiments such as "Excellent! Excellent!" The boys are singing loudly and very out of tune, and not together at all.

NARRATOR

The fact was, even though we sang harmonies that would make Quasimodo wince, chords not found in nature . . .

MS. HAYCOCK

(smiling and conducting nonstop) Good! Better!

NARRATOR

Nothing deterred Ms. Haycock. With a wisdom born of weeks of experience, she pushed on blindly, no, *deafly* toward a goal that was obviously beyond our grasp.

<end transcript>

The boys in the choir again put pressure on Kevin to say something to Ms. Haycock about not singing in the Spring Sing Concert, and he finally decides, "Aw, heck! Was I a stout-hearted man or a craven coward?" He speaks up during rehearsal and tells Ms. Haycock what the boys decided. On learning that "her boys" do not want to sing on the concert, Ms. Haycock turns away from the choir and begins to cry. Suddenly, the boys feel great remorse about Ms. Haycock's reaction and turn on Kevin.

<begin transcript>

IN THE CHOIR ROOM
Ms. Haycock is turned away from the choir, crying. The boys are all looking at each other with shock and horror and expressions of guilt.

NARRATOR

Needless to say, we handled it with a certain maturity.

EIGHTH-GRADE BOY 1 (to KEVIN)

Well, what'd you do that for, Kevin?!

KEVIN (to THE BOYS)

Me?! You told me to!

EIGHTH-GRADE BOY 2 (to KEVIN)

Way to go, Kev.

PAUL (to KEVIN)

I can't believe you did that.

EIGHTH-GRADE BOY 3 (to KEVIN)

You were supposed to talk to her! Not make her cry!

Ms. Haycock continues to cry.

NARRATOR

We had no idea what to do next. The only thing that could help us now was a miracle.

Ms. Haycock's crying becomes louder as her sobs increase. The boys look sad and unsure of what to do.

NARRATOR

And then, it happened.

Suddenly a high, sustained note can be heard. Someone is singing "Ahhhh" with a beautiful, clear, unchanged voice. It cuts through the crying and confusion, and all the boys look around to see where it is coming from. It is Warren Gander, who until now has not uttered a single sound or word. But now he has his mouth open wide, singing strong and clear and confident. The entire room turns toward him as Ms. Haycock stops crying and turns around as well.

NARRATOR

It took the tears of a student teacher to bring a song to the lips of Warren Gander.

While Warren holds the note on a long "Ahhh" the rest of the choir starts singing "Men, men, men, men, men . . ." and breaks out into "Stout-Hearted Men." Ms. Haycock's tears turn to a broad, bright smile.

NARRATOR

And the rest is history.

The boys are all singing, with Warren Gander's beautiful voice loudly and clearly guiding the rest of the group. The boys are all now singing pretty well in tune together with a great deal of zest and energy.

At this point, a professional recording of "Stout-Hearted Men" begins and we watch the eighth-grade boys singing all through their days: at school, on the bus, at home, carrying their music wherever they go.

NARRATOR

And so began the great Glee Club comeback of 1970! There were only two weeks before the big Spring Sing, but during those two weeks we breathed, slept, and ate "Stout-Hearted Men." It became our anthem, our battle cry, as we rallied around our secret weapon. It was kind of . . . infectious. And when the day finally arrived, we went from horrible to . . .

The professional recording suddenly cuts out and the boys are in their choir room, singing the final chord of "Stout-Hearted Men" as Ms. Haycock conducts. It is very loud and not in tune, but their level of enthusiasm is very high and Ms. Haycock is absolutely thrilled.

EIGHTH-GRADE BOYS' GLEE CLUB

(*singing*) . . . *MEN!!!*

MS. HAYCOCK

(grinning widely) Magnificent!!

NARRATOR

Well, anyway, we were ready.

AT THE SPRING SING CONCERT IN THE SCHOOL AUDITORIUM

The concert is under way and, when the scene opens, we can hear a women's choir on stage singing beautifully. The rest of the choirs are milling about backstage and comparing concert programs. Ms. Haycock arrives and excitedly passes out neckties for "her boys," who all put them on quietly as she speaks to them one more time before the performance.

MS. HAYCOCK

I am so proud of you all. Ever since I was a little girl . . .

NARRATOR

No, geez, don't tell us this! We don't wanna . . .

MS. HAYCOCK

. . . I've dreamed of standing up in front of a choir and molding them in song. Tonight will be my very first time and I have *you* to thank. *My men*. I'll never forget any of you.

NARRATOR

The funny thing is, in a way, that turned out to be true.

MS. HAYCOCK

Okay! Let's line up! We're next!

The boys walk onto the stage and take their places on the choral risers to sing "Stout-Hearted Men." Ms. Haycock then joins the choir on stage, bowing as the audience applauds before she steps in front of the boys.

NARRATOR

And so, from the murky depths of Mr. Frace's choir room, the eighth-grade boys' Glee Club finally stepped into the light. Sure we had misgivings.

But gazing down on Ms. Haycock's confident face, we knew we had nothing to fear. She *believed* in us. And, of course, we believed in Warren.

Ms. Haycock gives the boys reassuring smiles and then nods to the accompanist, and the piano opening to "Stout-Hearted Men" begins. The camera pans to different members of the choir, watching Ms. Haycock, looking nervous. Ms. Haycock is conducting a two pattern and the piano plays.

NARRATOR

But as I look back on that night, it isn't the anticipation that I remember best. And it isn't the faces in the audience.

Warren begins to sing a long, beautiful, high "ahhh" and Ms. Haycock smiles broadly and proudly at him, arm extended outward, encouraging his singing.

NARRATOR

What I remember best is that Warren Gander's voice chose *exactly that moment* . . .

Warren's voice cracks very loudly, and his beautiful, high "ahhh" clunks to a low, squeaky "awww." Ms. Haycock's face turns from joy to horror and surprise. The boys in the choir subtly turn and look at Warren, as well as each other. The audience members quietly look at one another.

NARRATOR

. . . to change.

Ms. Haycock gives a little smile and indicates to Warren to try again. Warren takes a deep breath and sings a beautiful, clear, high "Ahh" for a moment and then his voice loudly cracks and squeaks low. Warren's facial expression is one of confusion.

NARRATOR

It was *cruel*. In front of our very eyes, Warren had transformed from lyric tenor to . . .

Ms. Haycock gives Warren a third sign to begin again, but this time when he opens his mouth to sing, it is a low squeak and crack on "awww." He sounds like a frog croaking.

NARRATOR

. . . well, a bullfrog.

Audience members laugh quietly, but loudly enough to be heard. The boys suddenly turn restless on stage and start flipping through their music and looking at each other, unsure what to do.

NARRATOR

So the rest of us did the only thing we could. We panicked.

Ms. Haycock turns toward the pianist and whispers loudly, "Keep going!" The accompanist begins to play the opening of the song again.

MS. HAYCOCK

(whispering loudly to the choir) Keep going!

The boys are all looking in different places around the room, their faces looking confused and terrified. Some can be heard softly and unconfidently singing, "Men, men, men, men . . ." but all at different times. Some of them are not singing at all and flipping through their music, trying to figure out what to do. They, too, look confused and terrified.

NARRATOR

But the die was cast.

The boys' singing is getting louder and more chaotic-sounding. Lots of movement of the music results in lots of paper-shuffling noise. Paul begins sneezing uncontrollably from anxiety.

NARRATOR

Paul sneezed.
Which was too much for Doug.

Doug falls backwards off the risers and lands in a loud crash on the floor. The chaos on stage is growing and gaining volume quickly. Ms. Haycock is still conducting in a two pattern, which is growing more frantic by the moment.

NARRATOR

Somebody laughed. And I dropped my music.

MS. HAYCOCK

(whispering loudly and frantically as the song spirals out of control) Keep going!!

The boys are all singing loudly and at completely different times from one another. Someone tries to help Doug climb back onto the risers, but he falls again. The singing is getting louder and louder and less and less together. Paul keeps sneezing. Ms. Haycock is still conducting frantically.

NARRATOR

It was kind of a chain reaction. I'd like to say we rallied. But we didn't.

Ms. Haycock feverishly conducts a two pattern throughout the entire song. She ends with a big cut-off gesture, but many of the boys are buried in their music and continue to sing "Men, men, men . . ." until they realize they need to stop. Paul sneezes twice more in the silence. The camera shows many of the boys, including Warren Gander, who look at each other. They look more relieved that it is over than upset. Ms. Haycock looks absolutely numb.

NARRATOR

It was no one's fault, really, it's just that we had been pushed beyond our limits. We were a bunch of eighth-grade boys. Not an ensemble of stout-hearted men.

The audience applauds weakly and awkwardly. Ms. Haycock is clearly breathing heavily and turns to acknowledge the applause, with an exhausted and very upset look on her face. After she bows, she leaves the stage.

NARRATOR

As for Ms. Haycock, she dreamed of molding us into something we weren't. But that night, she got her wake-up call. The only problem was . . .

The boys extend their left arms toward the side of the stage where Ms. Haycock exited, as rehearsed, to give her an opportunity to return for another bow. The professional recording of "Stout Hearted-Men" from earlier in the episode begins to play. Ms. Haycock never reappears.

NARRATOR

. . . she wasn't there to answer.

While the boys freeze with their arms out to acknowledge their teacher, who is not coming back, Paul continues to sneeze uncontrollably. The music continues to play.

NARRATOR

We never found out where Ms. Haycock had disappeared to. Although some said she'd gone back to college.

Still, I'd like to think, wherever she is, there is a warm spot in her heart for the eighth-grade boys' Glee Club. After all, we'd learned together. And in a way, she'd learned from us. We'd learned together. Or so I like to tell myself.

Camera pans back to the school choir room where the episode began, where the boys are singing together, loudly and out of tune. Mr. Frace is standing at the window into the math classroom next door and, as the boys sing loudly, he closes the blinds in the window.

And Paul sneezes.

<end transcript>

The Goldbergs

The ABC sitcom *The Goldbergs* focuses on the Goldberg family during "1980-something" in Jenkintown, Pennsylvania. It is based on the real-life family of creator Adam F. Goldberg, who uses events from his upbringing as the foundation for each episode. In the show, Murray, the father (actor Jeff Garlin) is a furniture salesman, and Beverly (Wendi McLendon-Covey) is the stay-at-home mom whom all of her children refer to as "Smother" because of her incredibly overbearing nature. The oldest of the three children is Erica (Hayley Orrantia), who dreams of becoming a professional musician. Barry (Troy Gentile), the middle child, is bumbling and lovable, and—as a result of his Smother's overwhelming support and insistence that her children can do no wrong—believes that he is a master of karate and destined to be a professional basketball player someday. Adam, the youngest, is played by actor Sean Gambione; this character is the child version of the creator of the show. Two more characters are key: Grandpa (George Segal), known as Pops, often spends time at the Goldberg home, and the Narrator (voiced by Patton Oswalt) is supposed to be Adam F. Goldberg speaking retrospectively as an adult (as was done in *The Wonder Years*).

When the show began in 2013, Sean Gambione was approximately 14 years old in real life (the character Adam is intended to be a little younger than Sean in actuality) and he was physically small with an unchanged voice. As the show continued, Sean began to show real-life signs of puberty, including growth in height and heft and signifiers of voice change that included a change in the timbre of his speaking voice, some creaks and squeaks in his voice, and so forth. Most of these were not results of acting; it was clear that Sean was growing up. Instead of downplaying Sean's physiological changes through puberty, season three of *The Goldbergs* used this development and had Adam experience symptoms of puberty alongside Sean. For example, in the episode "Couples Costume" (season 3, episode 6) Adam and Erica are talking about Adam's Halloween plans with his girlfriend. She is telling him that he and his girlfriend are no longer children:

<begin transcript>

ERICA

You are adults now. Just listen to your deep, yet still . . . high . . .weird voice.

ADAM

(*in a naturally higher but not childlike voice*) Hurtful. But continue.

<end transcript>

In the episode "In Conclusion, Thanksgiving" (season 3, episode 8), Adam's uncle Marvin has just arrived for the holiday. He is filling Adam in on all that he has been doing lately:

<begin transcript>

UNCLE MARVIN

I'm feelin' good! I lost 10 pounds. Gained 6, lost 4, gained 2. Also, your voice is weird.

ADAM

(*in a naturally higher, not childlike, thin voice and a resigned tone*) It is. I'm . . . I'm hoping this isn't where it lands.

UNCLE MARVIN

(enthusiastically) Ha ha! That's the spirit!

<end transcript>

As a child of the 1980s and 1990s, I think this show is genius in its portrayals of pop culture of the time period. Moreover, the characters are fantastic and I adore each in his or her own way—knowing that so much of them is based on fact makes them that much more endearing. The writing is intelligent and funny on multiple levels and, as an advocate for adolescents, I especially enjoyed the way the show portrayed Adam in season three as he experienced puberty. It was genuine and sincere. One episode in particular, "A Chorus Lie" (season 3, episode 2) specifically focuses on Adam's love of singing in middle school and his changing voice:

<begin transcript>

Film clips of Adam as a young, adorable boy roll past as the narrator sets the scene.

NARRATOR

Back in the day, I was a *ridiculously* cute kid. I'm not bragging, it's just pure fact. But of course, no one stays a kid forever . . .

It is apparent that we are now in the present day in the Goldbergs' bathroom. Adam is looking in the mirror as his brother, Barry, applies an enormous bandage to Adam's chin.

ADAM

(*looking concerned*) Are you sure about this? People are gonna know that I'm covering up a zit.

BARRY

Don't worry, pal. I'll just tell everyone I pummeled your face.

ADAM

(*smiling*) You're a good brother.

BARRY

The best! Here, you have a giant one forming on your forehead too. (*Barry snaps a huge pair of skiing goggles onto Adam's forehead to cover up his forming pimple.*)

The scene switches to the middle school gymnasium, where Adam and his classmates are sitting on little yellow scooters and racing across the floor, pushing themselves and passing a ball with their feet.

NARRATOR

Maybe I could hide the pimples, but the rest was hard to mask.

COACH MELLOR

Come on, hustle! This is "scooter" ball! Not "sit in the corner and talk to Kevin" ball!

NARRATOR

I began to smell different . . .

Adam coasts in front of Coach Mellor, who reacts strongly as Adam passes by.

COACH MELLOR

(*gasping, horrified*) WHOA! GOLDFARB! Wheel it in!!

Adam backs up to Coach so they can talk.

COACH MELLOR

Time for a private huddle. I'm going to put this delicately, kid. You smell like a gym sock's butt.

ADAM

Um, thanks.

COACH MELLOR

You smell like a garlic diaper.

ADAM

Thanks?

COACH MELLOR

You smell like egg salad left in a humidifier.

ADAM

(*annoyed*) Thanks.

COACH MELLOR

I assume that you don't notice since you live with that stink 24-7.

ADAM

(*looking defeated and matter-of-fact*) Oh, no, I smell it.

COACH MELLOR

Listen, I have a Speed Stick® in my desk. It's yours now. Be liberal with it. Coach is on your team here. That's why I pulled you aside to avoid embarrassment.

ADAM

I guess I wish you could have pulled me aside just a *little farther*.

The camera pans out and all of Adam's classmates have rolled up around them on their scooters and are listening intently to the conversation between Coach and him.

NARRATOR

I was eating like an animal and suddenly seeing *every* woman I came across in a new light.

Murray Goldberg walks into the room where Adam is wolfing down a big bowl of cereal and watching television.

MURRAY

Have you seen my *TV Guide* with Sally Jessy Raphael on the cover?

ADAM

Uh-uh. Nope. (*As his dad leaves the room, Adam sheepishly pulls the missing issue of* TV Guide *out from under a couch pillow.*)

NARRATOR

Every woman.

ADAM

(*staring at Sally Jesse Raphael with a lusty look on his face)* Man oh man. Those looks *and* emotional intelligence to boot? Wow.

NARRATOR

But worst of all, it affected my *favorite* activity in the world! *The annual school musical.*

The camera pans to Adam walking into the music classroom where his middle school music teacher, Miss Cinoman, is seated behind the piano. The sheet music for the song "I Can Do That" from the Broadway musical *A Chorus Line* is propped up on the music stand.

MISS CINOMAN

(*warmly*) Welcome, Mr. Goldberg! I have a feeling that *this* might finally be the year that you break out of the chorus!

Miss Cinoman plays a few opening chords of "I Can Do That." Adam sings along with her, full of enthusiasm, but quite out of tune.

ADAM

I'm watchin' Sis go pitter pat, Said,
"I can do that."
"I can do that!"

Miss Cinoman puts up her hand quickly to signal Adam to stop singing. The look on her face is one of discomfort.

NARRATOR

Turns out, I could *not do that.*

MISS CINOMAN

(*choosing her words very* carefully) Well . . . you, um . . . . you *really* (*pause*) really *sang* it. You sang it.

ADAM

I know in past years I was upset when you put me in the chorus, but I'm thinking *this year* it feels *right.*

MISS CINOMAN

(*excited*) *Done!* You're in the chorus!

ADAM

(*relieved, throwing head back)* Oh, *thank God!*

MISS CINOMAN

Chorus *Line*, which is *a lead*!

ADAM

(*confused*) But I'm in the chorus?

MISS CINOMAN

(*excited*) *Line!*

ADAM

(*relieved again*) Oh, thank *God*!

MISS CINOMAN

(*excited*) Which means you have a big solo!

ADAM

But I'm in the chorus . . .

MISS CINOMAN

(*excited*) *Line!*

ADAM

(*confused*) But did you not hear the . . . sounds I just made?

MISS CINOMAN

Adam, every boy your age sounds like you. And honestly, I don't have that much to work with here, so I might as well just give the leads to the most enthusiastic kids.

ADAM

(*looking horrified; in a soft voice*) Balls.

MISS CINOMAN

(*looking defeated*) Yeah. Balls.
(*excited again*) Okay! Let's take it from the top! Sing it with me!

ADAM

(*singing in a different key from the piano*) *I'm watchin' Sis go pitter pat . . .*

MISS CINOMAN

(*trying to sing with Adam*) Try to stay in the key.

ADAM

(*starting over, singing more loudly, but again singing in a different key from the piano*) *I'm watchin' Sis go pitter pat . . .*

MISS CINOMAN

(*again, trying to sing with Adam*) You are kind of all over the map. Okay.
(*singing for Adam, modeling the right key and notes*) *I'm watchin' Sis go pitter pat . . .*

ADAM

(*singing largely out of tune*) *"I can do that!"*

MISS CINOMAN

(*looking horrified, but trying to hide it*) You know, it's mostly a dance show and you bring a lot of dance energy.

(*looking off to the side, defeated; quiet voice*) Balls.

<end transcript>

As the episode "A Chorus Lie" continues, Adam returns home horrified that he has been given a lead in the school musical. The following conversation ensues:

<begin transcript>

Adam walks through the front door and Beverly and Pops are seated at the dining room table, playing cards. Beverly smiles broadly at her son as he walks in.

BEVERLY

There's my tiny snuggle angel!

ADAM

(*angrily*) *Stop it!* I'm not tiny. Or snuggly. Or angel-y!

POPS

(*surprised*) Tough day at the office, kiddo?

ADAM

The worst! I got the lead in the musical!

BEVERLY

(*excited*) Schmoo! That's fantastic! That's all you've ever wanted!

ADAM

(*sadly and quietly*) *Not* any more.
My face is breaking out.
My pits are stinky.
And my voice is very, *very* unpredictable.
I *finally* get the part of a lifetime and I'm just going to humiliate myself.

POPS

Ah yes! The wondrous journey through puberty!

ADAM

(sadly) It's not wondrous. It's *awful*.

<end transcript>

Adam's mother contemplates his journey through what the Goldberg family refers to as "The Pubening" and decides that she can help him navigate puberty so smoothly that it will be like he skipped right over it, and also a little *fun*. Pops objects and warns her that you cannot skip puberty and that her plan is a bad idea. Beverly disregards the warning and takes Adam to the Gimbels makeup counter, where he is given a makeover with foundation and powder.

<begin transcript>

ADAM

(*at the Gimbels makeup counter, looking happily into the mirror at his, now, flawless complexion*) What kind of sorcery is this?! My giant zits are *gone*!

BEVERLY

Mama made you a promise! Now your adorable punim is ready to light up that stage!

NARRATOR

Just one problem. My singing voice. My mom couldn't fix that. That is . . . until some news broke that shook the country . . .

<end transcript>

This show pulled in real pop culture happenings from the 1980s and early 1990s throughout every episode. At this point in this particular episode, the Narrator tells the viewers the tale of Milli Vanilli, one of the most popular international pop acts of the time. They sold millions of albums worldwide, but it turned out that they actually never recorded their own voices and they lip-synced all performances. It was truly a scandal in real life, and those of you old enough to remember it will likely never forget the ridiculousness. The members of Milli Vanilli were stripped of their Grammy for Best New Artist and immediately solidified their infamy, not as musicians, but as a shameful lip-syncing duo.

Later in the day, after Adam's Gimbels makeover, Beverly and Adam are watching the news at home and learn about the Milli Vanilli scandal. Suddenly, Beverly gets the idea that Adam could lip-sync his performance for *A Chorus Line* and bypass concerns about his voice change altogether.

BEVERLY

(*very excited*) Problem solved, lovebug!! We're gonna Milli Vanilli the f**k out of that musical!!

Now armed with a plan, Beverly and Adam meet with Miss Cinoman, the music teacher to propose a strategy.

<begin transcript>

The scene opens in Miss Cinoman's middle school music classroom, where she is seated at her desk; a trombone can be seen behind her, maracas are scattered across her desk, and her lamp is made from the neck an upright string bass. Beverly and Adam take a seat at her desk, across from her.

NARRATOR

My mom's plan for me only needed to get past one person for it to succeed.

BEVERLY

Susan, I really appreciate you agreeing to see me on such short notice.

MISS CINOMAN

Technically, I didn't agree. You just barged in during third period and yelled "class dismissed."

BEVERLY

Point is, I understand you are putting together a cast for this year's musical and it's presented some . . . challenges.

MISS CINOMAN

(*looking completely disgusted*) It's a real suck show.

(*turning quickly to Adam, smiling*) You're gonna be . . . great!

ADAM

(*smiling*) I won't be, but that's sweet to say.

BEVERLY

Well, what if I had a way to solve your problems? A way to make this your biggest hit yet!

MISS CINOMAN

(*looking exasperated*) Mrs. Goldberg, we have been through this in the past. You *can't* be in the musical.

BEVERLY

No, no, no, I've come to accept that. I'm talking about a different approach *entirely.* Have you heard of this Milli Vanilli scandal?

MISS CINOMAN

Big fan. (*choking up*) Hit me hard.

BEVERLY

(*sympathetically*) I'm sorry. But what if someone could do the same thing only without making the same sloppy mistakes?

MISS CINOMAN

(*surprised*) Are you actually suggesting that Adam lip sync his songs in the show?

BEVERLY

(*quietly*) God, I guess hearing it out loud it really does sound insane, even for me . . .

MISS CINOMAN

(*excited and animated*) *Screw it!* I'm in!

ADAM

(*surprised*) Really?

MISS CINOMAN

I'll get all the kids to do it! I mean, what choice do I have?!

BEVERLY

(*very excited*) None! Yay!

MISS CINOMAN

(*also very excited*) Yay!

ADAM

(*in a very high, squeaky, excited voice*) Yay!!

Beverly and Miss Cinoman look at Adam in horror.

BEVERLY (to ADAM)

Mouth it! (*Beverly then says "Yay!" while Adam lip syncs her voice.*)

<end transcript>

Adam works on his performance and tries out the song "I Can Do That" for Pops, but really is lip-syncing to a professional recording of the show while attempting to tap dance. At first Pops doesn't realize that Adam is lip-syncing and is completely amazed, saying, "This is *incredible!* My grandson's a superstar!" That is, until the recording skips in place and it becomes clear that Adam was not actually singing.

<begin transcript>

POPS

So, wait . . . you actually weren't doing anything?

ADAM

Not doing anything?! Did you see this?! (*begins to break out into the tap dancing routine that accompanied the song*)

POPS (to BEVERLY)

(*upset*) Bevy, you can't let him go through with this cockamamie scheme!

BEVERLY

(*proud*) Well, actually, it was *my* idea.

POPS

Oh, God. Why?!

ADAM

Pops, I can't go on stage and completely embarrass myself!

POPS

(*upset and confused*) Just do your best! You're the same great kid you always were.

ADAM

(*sad and frustrated, in a squeaky voice, with a very defeated look on his face*) Listen to me! Do I *sound* like the same kid?! Do I *look* like the same kid?! NO! I'm not him. I'm . . . . *whatever* this is. And if Mom can make it better, I'm gonna let her. (*Adam leaves the room, clicking away sadly in his tap shoes.*)

BEVERLY

(*looking at Pops, who is giving her a sad look*) Don't give me that look. As his mother it is my job to make this all better.

POPS

But you can't. All you're *doing* is making it worse. You're turning him into something he's not.

Adam angrily clicks back into the room in his tap shoes and picks up a powder-blue Caboodle carrier from the table next to the stereo.

ADAM

I forgot my foundation, rouge, and powder puff! Good day to you, sir. (*angrily click-stomps away*)

IMMEDIATE SCENE CHANGE

Backstage at the middle school, right before show time for *A Chorus Line*. Adam and his friends are all lined up in front of Miss Cinoman, who is standing next to a big tape deck.

NARRATOR

The biggest night of my middle school musical theater career had arrived, and the only one who was more nervous than me was my Smother.

MISS CINOMAN

Okay! Let's warm up! I have the recording of the New York City Boys Choir doing scales, so show me what you've got.

Miss Cinoman presses "play" on the tape deck and a professional recording of young male voices singing solfège scales begins, "Do, re, mi, fa, sol . . ." Adam and his castmates begin to mouth each of the syllables along with the recorded voices. Beverly is standing off to the side of the room, looking upset.

MISS CINOMAN

Oh, very good! Very good! *Move those lips!* No sounds!

NARRATOR

Watching us Milli Vanilli our way through the warmup scales, my mom realized Pops was right.

BEVERLY

(*approaching Miss Cinoman*) Susan, we need to talk.

MISS CINOMAN

Sorry, show starts in five.

BEVERLY

No, you can't do this. It's wrong and you know it.

MISS CINOMAN

(*frustrated*) What are you talking about? This whole thing was all *your idea*!

BEVERLY

Those people out there, they want to see *A Chorus Line,* not *A Chorus Lie.*

MISS CINOMAN

(*irritated*) I'm so confused by your moral high ground. Again, this was all you!

ADAM

Mom, it's fine! (*happily)* This recording is going to blow the frickin' roof off this place!

BEVERLY (TO THE ENTIRE CAST)

And so will you, with your own voices! Yes, they are creaking and cracking and, yes, your foreheads are *very* shiny. All right? And you take insanely--long-showers. *But it doesn't matter!* Because you're all just as amazing as you *always* were.

ADAM

(*looking sad and frustrated*) I don't *feel* amazing.

FRIEND DAVE KIM

(*looking very annoyed*) *You*?! What's your problem?

ADAM

(*in a squeaky high voice*) *Oh,* you heard my voice . . .

DAVE KIM

Who cares?! I got "bacne," dude. *Crazy* bacne.

FRIEND #2

(*looking at Dave Kim*) So?! I sweat *constantly* for no reason. (*looking around*) I'm sweating right now and it's, like, 50 degrees in here!

FRIEND #3

(*looking horrified*) I've got a weird thing for Sally Jesse Raphael. (*Upon hearing this, Adam gets a funny look on his face.*)

BEVERLY

See? None of you are alone! You're all going through something that *everybody* has to suffer through. Come on! Who's with me?

MISS CINOMAN

(*confidently*) Screw it! Let's go out there and give them the *best worst* musical the school has ever seen!

NARRATOR

And so we sang it. *We really sang it.* And it wasn't pretty. But it was *definitely us.*

The music begins to play for the song "Kiss Today Goodbye" from *A Chorus Line*. Adam has the opening solo and is singing it with heart, confidence, and a very wobbly, squeaky, thin, sincere voice. His friends join him in singing, and they all sound wobbly and cracking but glorious in their own way. Beverly and Pops are watching from the audience, emotional and proud.

ADAM

Kiss today goodbye
The sweetness and the sorrow

FULL COMPANY

(*wobbly singing, sincere*) *Wish me luck, the same to you . . .*

NARRATOR

Sure, growing up is hard and awkward and embarrassing. But if you're lucky, you just might find the courage to sing your way through it.

FULL COMPANY

What I did for love . . . (We hear wobbly, unstable falsetto and voices an octave below. Pops has a forced smile on his face as he listens, and Beverly is throwing little kisses to Adam on stage.)

<end transcript>

DISTILLATION

These television episodes are from three different eras that collectively span more than forty years, yet the message remained the same: voice change is hard and embarrassing, and adolescents generally do not feel good about the process. Although forty years is a long period of time, it is a drop in the bucket of the decades during which many people have maintained an embittered way of thinking about the changing voice. We cannot alter past viewpoints, but we certainly can influence perspectives moving forward. What follows is a distillation of the above episodes with supporting discussion to expose deep-rooted views about voice change and puberty. As you read, I encourage you to consider how we might counterbalance these views through our work as music educators and our advocacy for adolescents.

Self-Perception

Portrayal of the changing voice in these television episodes is pretty accurate in that the voice can be unpredictable, all sounds are not conventionally pretty, and vocal challenges proceed on their own timeline. However, when the characters call themselves "losers" or say that "they stink" or that they "don't feel amazing," twinges of melancholy tug at my heartstrings. Popular television shows capitalize on the frustrations of voice change, keeping negativity as the core of the experience. As stated earlier in this book, the changing voice is not always the prettiest sound, but it is incredibly sincere and honest. It has to be celebrated for what it *is*, not mourned for what it *isn't*, especially by the singers themselves.

There should be no reason why our students feel like losers because of their voice change (unless they use the term in reference to actually losing their children's voice, but I think that's reaching a bit). We teach choral students for multiple years, so we can easily reinforce the idea of adolescents' voice change as a holistic, full-self experience that is larger than merely the quality of their vocal sounds. In addition, choral music education is flush with opportunities for fostering feelings of pride and developing communities of support, which are key elements in perseverance through voice change. Adolescent singers need to see themselves as positive contributors to the larger mission, whether or not they are singing in tune. They need to understand that we are proud of them when they make genuine efforts, when they are *trying*. It is also essential that they understand what is and what is not within their control and celebrate small but significant accomplishments. More than anything, adolescents should understand that they are not losers because they are not losing at anything; rather, they are succeeding as they are growing and developing just as they are supposed to. In *The Goldbergs*, Adam said that he didn't "feel amazing." How might we have helped him feel better about himself if he was in our choral program?

The featured character in all three of the quoted episodes worried about failing someone because of voice change. In *The Brady Bunch*, Peter says, "I don't want to let the others down" in reference to his siblings. The overly enthusiastic student teacher in *The Wonder Years*, Ms. Haycock, gives a pre-performance talk about her now-realized dream of working with a choir and her pride in her "men." This concerns Kevin, who wonders about how things are actually going to play out during the performance; none of the boys wants to let her down. Adam in *The Goldbergs* is most concerned about embarrassing himself and letting himself down, bringing in the role of the invisible audience during voice change; more on this in a moment. It's as if the characters internalize the idea of being *broken* because their voices were changing: There is something wrong with me and, as a result, I am going to inadvertently ruin something for someone else.

A good way to counterbalance this thinking is, first and foremost, to honor where each student is in the voice change process and help all of them feel good about the genuine efforts they are putting forth—regardless of how pretty or in tune the sound may be. It is also important to acknowledge that, yes, this is really tricky right now, but you (the teacher) are proud of the efforts the students are making. Practically speaking, students can turn their focus to aspects of the music that can be manipulated apart from pitches, keeping the emphasis on rhythms, vitality, emotion, diction, text expression, exploration of registers, stance and breathing, and so forth; there is much that students can feel positive about. As they do what they *can* do, also encourage levity throughout the process, especially when voices do not operate as desired or intended. The bottom line is that our work should bellow that adolescents are *not* losers because of voice change. They are perfectly normal and fantastic and still capable of great things. The bigger picture is that control of the voice *will* improve as students grow and all the parts of the larynx coordinate again.

Choral Music Educators

As the old adage goes, "If you can't stand the heat, get out of the kitchen." With regard to working with adolescents and changing voices, many choral teachers are glorious Julia Childs in the kitchen, but others cannot stand the heat. I have met music teachers like Mr. Frace in *The Wonder Years* who are horrified at the sound of the changing voice and who would rather negotiate an hour of silent study hall than work with changing voices. I have also met those like Ms. Haycock, who initially oozed enthusiasm for "her boys," but her unrealistic expectations and focus on personal glory resulted in her ultimately leaving her choir because they sang poorly in their concert. These fictional teachers were not good fits for working with changing voices and there are real-life choral teachers who operate in the same ways. These portrayals are problematic if accepted as the overarching attitude of choral music educators toward adolescent singers.

Miss Cinoman in *The Goldbergs* is another interesting representation of a music educator. She clearly enjoys working with her students, although some of her efforts are a bit misguided. I like her because she thinks in ways that are seemingly realistic for actual middle school choral teachers, such as when she says, "Adam, every boy your age sounds like you. And honestly, I don't have that much to work with here, so I might as well just give the leads to the most enthusiastic kids." The concern with the character is that Miss Cinoman says things out loud that should never be said to students. Although choral teachers may have thoughts similar to those of Miss Cinoman, such as "It's a real suck show" or "Let's go out there and give them the best worst musical the school has ever seen!" (which is part of the reason her character is so funny), these sorts of comments should never actually be said to students. If middle school students heard you describe their performance as a "suck show" it could hurt them deeply (especially if they look up to you) and they could stop singing altogether. My concern about the way Miss Cinoman is portrayed is that she will lead people to think it is more acceptable to reveal such sentiments to adolescents, especially with regard to their changing voice.

Stay with me for a related story: The television show *House* was a hit series during its run from 2004 to 2012. It focused on the work of a doctor named Gregory House (actor Hugh Laurie) who was brilliant but also bitter, antisocial, and unorthodox. I loved the show and watched every episode. At some point during its run, I had a conversation about *House* with my father, whose career in healthcare led him to interact with doctors on a regular basis. He did not like the show because of the way House treated other people, especially his patients and medical team. According to my father's experiences, such portrayals—especially those that become really popular—made it more socially acceptable for doctors to speak down to or ridicule patients: that is how they are portrayed on television, so it must be okay. At the time I did not really get what he was saying and was left wondering, "People would not stand for such treatment, right?.." But now I understand his point. Portrayals of middle school choral teachers such as Mr. Frace and Miss Cinoman might be people's only source of information about how a music teacher interacts with students whose voices are changing, and if so, the way these fictional characters interact becomes an accepted norm within the voice change simulacrum.

The Invisible Audience

The episode of *The Goldbergs* couched voice change within the larger picture of puberty, evident in the opening pastiche of adolescence. Not only was Adam's voice changing, he was smelling differently, considering females in new ways, eating more, and so on. The writers included the idea of the invisible audience in his story arc and throughout the entire episode, as Adam was hyperfocused on his changing voice and how mortifying it would be to crack in front of others while singing. Put your hand up close to your face for Adam's perspective—all that he could see was about *him*, all that he did was to protect *him* from the ridicule of others, and he blindly listened to his mother, who said that she could make puberty better for *him*. At the end of the episode, when Adam made his comment to his class about not feeling amazing, suddenly the bigger picture was much clearer. His friends did not care about *his* changing voice because they were too concerned with their own puberty to care about Adam's cracking voice. Adam's perception that his peers would judge him and think less of him because of his changing voice were unfounded; in reality, no one was paying much attention to him at all. That invisible audience was a powerful presence for Adam and contributed to feelings of insecurity and fear of singing, but his fears were unfounded.

Our choral students are influenced by the invisible audience, and how that audience is perceived at a given moment impacts adolescents' well-being. We cannot destroy the invisible audience for our students, but we *can* encourage our adolescent singers to share their experiences and insights regarding music, text, voice change challenges, social justice, anything that provides the chance to have a voice among their peers and hear what others their age are experiencing. Anything we can do to pull that hypothetical hand away from their faces and broaden students' perspectives about themselves and the larger world is well worth the effort. With a bigger picture of their voices, the music, the voice change process, and those around them comes increased willingness to try new musical things, sing out, persevere through vocal challenges, enjoy their voice a little more, and perhaps occasionally disregard the invisible audience.

Unpredictability and Others

Vocal unpredictability is prevalent in the storylines of all three episodes. It is especially poignant that, not only do the featured characters have negative reactions to their vocal unpredictability, but people close to them express negative emotions about it. In *The Brady Bunch*, Greg tries to help Peter's voice "sound like it used to," resorting to home remedies of water, steam, and honey. Peter himself tries to "scream [his] voice" back to pre–voice change quality and function. Despite all attempts, Peter's voice is changing and there is nothing anyone can do about it. Not only is he quite upset about all of this, his siblings are equally upset and torn about what to do with him, especially Greg: should they keep him in their singing group or exclude him because he might "mess up" their sound? In *The Wonder Years*, Warren Gander's sudden voice change ultimately results in all sorts of performance chaos and Ms. Haycock's disappearing forever, even though she had finally fulfilled her dream of "molding [a choir] in song." During *The Goldbergs*, the main characters and music teacher are willing to allow the students to lip-sync an entire musical soundtrack to avoid the unpredictability of their voices because, as Miss Cinoman says, "What choice do I have?"

Unpredictability is a natural part of the voice change process and is best traversed whole-heartedly by both the choral teacher and the singers. Vocal surprises are unavoidable, but not unembraceable. As the famous children's book *We're Going on a Bear Hunt* repeatedly exclaims:

> We can't go over it!
> We can't go under it!
> Oh no! We've got to go through it! (Rosen, 1989)

When unpredictable vocal moments are embraced as a natural and inevitable part of voice change, student fear and trepidation are reduced. It is also necessary to give reassurance that the student will not be abandoned or shamed by family, friends, or the teacher as a result of such moments. Adam in *The Goldbergs* understood that his voice is "very, *very* unpredictable," which fostered fear about what could potentially come out of his mouth while singing and fear of how people would react. Yes, this is a fictional show, but this fear is very real for adolescents experiencing voice change, so much so that unpredictability of the voice influences many adolescents to stop singing altogether during this time of their lives. My choral teacher friend, Deb Borton, constantly worked to calm her middle school singers' fears:

> We understand how important and how precious it is when somebody has the guts. And I'll tell them, "I don't care if a small ferret flies out of your throat, nobody's going to laugh at you. Even if it looks darn funny if a ferret flies out of your throat, we're not laughing." (Sweet, 2016a, p. 80)

Easing students' fears involves providing information about what is happening with their voices, helping them realize what they can and cannot manipulate at various moments, reinforcing that voice change is not a forever experience, and reassuring students that we are *all* in this together and I, your choral teacher, will always have your back.

Closing Thoughts About the Episodes

When I watch these three episodes, of course I laugh! The writing is smart and funny and the delivery is fantastic throughout. And wow, can that Peter Brady crack his voice *on cue*. As I transcribed these episodes for this chapter, my two small children often hung around to watch the process. While I know that these are funny shows and that they have some threads of positivity woven into them, the general idea of each was that voice change was really unpleasant. My children asked me, "Mom, what is happening to him?" and I found myself responding, "His voice is changing. It happens to everyone. It will happen to you someday," and then I realized that I did not want them to think that their voice change experiences would necessarily be like those of the characters in these television shows. We talked about why the voice changes, how it can be tricky, and the positive outcomes of the experience. The conversations I had with my children balanced what they saw in the episodes. If they only watched these episodes with no follow-up discussion, their understandings of voice change would likely be rooted in impressions of fear, embarrassment, and unpredictability well before they got to middle school. They saw boys being really embarrassed by their voices; this is not what I want my son and daughter to think about their singing voices at any point in life.

My interactions with my own children demonstrated exactly what I want to say in this chapter: pop culture and mainstream portrayals of voice change have great power to perpetuate understanding *and* misunderstanding of voice change for adolescents, even before they reach puberty. Choral music educators are not immune from the power of pop culture influence, either. My work has taken me to many conferences over the years, and I always have conversations with music educators who feel dread, fear, and frustration about the adolescent changing voice. Many of them have never worked with the changing voice before. Where do these strong emotions come from? If they have no experience working with the changing voice, why do they feel so negatively about it? I am not placing blame for negative perceptions of adolescent voice change on the backs of *The Brady Bunch, The Wonder Years*, or *The Goldbergs,* especially because these are only three of many portrayals of the experience (see the Additional Resources section for a few more examples). What I am saying is that if children and developing adolescents, as well as developing choral music educators, are continually steeped in mostly glass-half-empty perceptions of the voice change experience and adolescence, people will likely foster negative perceptions before encounters with voice change (or adolescents) ever occur.

Here is where the idea of the simulacrum comes back into play. Our situated reality with regard to voice change, both as a profession and as part of the larger society, is established and limited by our understandings and misunderstandings of adolescence and voice change. As pop culture portrayals continue to reinforce the experience as one of turmoil and negativity, the voice change simulacrum will preserve a bleak perspective of adolescence and the changing voice. Without conscious efforts to transform the narrative, this negative simulacrum will continue to impact the choral music education profession for years to come.

DIGEST

Advocating for the Changing Voice

Many choral educators and advocates of adolescent voice change are already working to counteract negative thinking about the changing voice. I applaud *every* effort to initiate positive ripples with students, families, colleagues, and leaders in the choral profession. Keep up the great work! I also greatly appreciate initiatives within professional organizations to validate changing voices as worthy and important and not as something broken. What follow are brief highlights of three choirs that overtly support their adolescent members as they experience voice change and work to keep them as part of the larger professional organization.

The Chicago Children's Choir (https://ccchoir.org/) created DiMension, a choir specifically for young men with changing or changed voices in elementary, middle, and high school. The CCC website describes DiMension:

> Singers learn to understand their own voices through male ensemble singing, solo opportunities, sight reading, and music theory. Training and repertoire are specifically designed to guide young men through the vocal transition, while learning to sing a diverse repertoire with musicality, movement and expression.

The Pacific Boychoir Academy (www.pacificboychoir.org) in Oakland, California, includes the following statement on its website:

> By design and necessity, Pacific Boychoir music staff are experts in boys' changing voices, how to use them without hurting them. As the proverb goes that, "if you can speak, you can sing," we believe that anybody who can speak has notes they can use to sing. Training changing boys' voices means having a willingness to monitor constantly shifting voices, changing voice parts as needed, and picking individual notes or phrases to modify. This kind of care allows teenagers in the Pacific Boychoir to continue to sing throughout their high school years. (Branded name vocal training, http://www.pacificboychoir.org/day-school/troubadors)

The Wilten Boys' Choir (www.saengerknaben.com), centered in Innsbruck, Austria, is recognized as one of the finest musical ensembles in Europe, dating back to the 13th century. Much support is in place within the organization to help singers through the challenges of voice change. The following comes from an interview with Johannes Stecher, who began as artistic director of the Wilten Boys' Choir in 1991.

> A note on changed voices: "This is not a disease. In the past, boys did not rehearse or perform while their voices were changing. I don't think that singing while the voice is changing can lead to bad habits and injuries. Even after their voices break, the boys continue to be voice-trained by highly qualified singing tutors. In the last 25 years, many former members of the choir went on to become successful singers, musicians and music educators. Boys whose voices change may remain in the ensemble singing in their new range. Vocally, the boys are encouraged to continue to learn healthy singing; when the boy's voice will begin to change, individual instruction may be necessary to aid him through the transition. Boys continue to hone their skills—and stay in the choir until they go to University or until they marry and settle down." (Fabienne, 2016, https://www.blog.tirol/en/2016/12/ethereal-voices-from-tirol-the-wilten-boys-choir/)

Although these are only three brief examples, it is heartening to know that there are active efforts in place to challenge the voice change simulacrum where adolescent singers are honored and encouraged to continue singing during and after voice change, well into adulthood and throughout the rest of their lives.

Female Voice Change in Pop Culture

Although research has proved that voice change is experienced by female and male adolescents, I cannot recall overt acknowledgment of female voice change in a pop culture venue. Female voice change is largely not acknowledged within music education and the broader society, so it is not surprising that this phenomenon has not carried over into television, movies, and books. You can hear scant examples of the female changing voice in pop culture if you open an ear to them. One is the song "Do You Want to Build a Snowman?" from the 2013 Disney animated movie *Frozen*. If you listen carefully to the differences between the three singers who portray Anna in this song, you can detect three different stages of the female voice. Katie Lopez was the voice of Anna at age five and her voice is clear and clean, clearly a child's voice. Agatha Lee Monn portrayed Anna as a nine-year-old, and though she sings in a lovely way, her voice is raspier than that of five-year old Anna. She reaches a little for higher notes, suggesting slight challenges in her upper range; her tone also has less color than does that of the younger singer. Veteran actress Kristen Bell voiced Anna at age 18, and her voice is that of a fully developed woman. Her sound is strong and clear, full and colorful, and her voice is nuanced with vibrato. She has great control of her voice and demonstrates a wide vocal range.

Additional media portrayals of female voice change have been extremely difficult to find, but further examples of the male changing voice in television or movies are provided in the Additional Resources section at the end of this book.

CHAPTER 5
Exploring Eminent Perspectives

I have great respect for the past. If you don't know where you've come from, you don't know where you're going. I have respect for the past, but I'm a person of the moment. I'm here, and I do my best to be completely centered at the place I'm at, then I go forward to the next place.

Maya Angelou

The past is a great place and I don't want to erase it or to regret it, but I don't want to be its prisoner either.

Mick Jagger

I advocate for approaching adolescent changing voices on a case-by-case basis and believe that the process of voice change is not predetermined, nor is the outcome. In conversations with fellow choral educators, I have found that most also agree that adolescents progress through voice change at their own pace, in their own way, with their own results. What is curious to me, then, is the intensity of focus on classification of adolescent singers in the larger choral profession. My own preference aligns with music education professor Patrick Freer's commentary on the chicken-and-the-egg nature of this matter:

> We do not seek to understand the changing voice through voice classifications. Rather, the classifications result from our understanding of the changing voice. Classifications are only helpful if they can assist us in selecting repertoire, choosing pedagogical techniques, and knowing what characteristics we can expect from these boys and their voices in the months and years to come. (2010, p. 33)

I celebrate Freer's perspective, but I am not convinced that these sentiments are shared by the majority of the choral profession. A very truthful disclaimer: I am not anti-voice classification system. I greatly appreciate the work that has been done in this area and understand thoroughly that the systems were designed to help students and teachers. What I struggle with is the way these systems are upheld as the key to working with the changing voices. Adolescents are growing, changing, and developing across the board. Because rapid and unpredictable growth is taking place inside and outside the entire body, from the larynx down to cellular levels, there is no *one* classification system that will cleanly map out the voice change of all of our students, whether female or male. I acknowledge that the respected systems may provide insight into where the voice could potentially go during voice change, so in that respect they can help ease some of the fear associated with the changing voice. Yet voice change is bigger than classification, and conversations need to include physiological, psychological, and emotional considerations if we are to holistically assist and validate adolescent singers during this time in their life.

In the movie *Pirates of the Caribbean* (Verbinski, 2003) there is discussion of a pirate code that dictates the conduct of the pirates aboard the fictional ship the *Black Pearl*. Apparently pirate codes were real, and preserved documents have provided details about rules of discipline, division of stolen goods, compensation for injured pirates, and so forth. In the movie, Captain Barbosa (actor Geoffrey Rush) ultimately admits that instead of being absolute and unwavering, "the code is more guidelines, than actual rules." I support a similar shift of thinking in the choral music profession: so that voice classification systems are used more as guidelines for helping teachers assist adolescent singers through voice change than as steadfast stages through which all voices pass; so that the systems are utilized as supporting tools to help guide the process of voice change rather than label adolescent singers' changing voices; so that social media formats encourage awareness and wellness of the entire singer as best practice for teaching adolescents instead of automatically recommending that voices be sorted into categories; and so that we, as Freer (2010) said, consider the students' voices first.

With reference to the discussion of simulacrum in chapter 4, when new choral professionals enter the field they are quickly socialized by the endorsed practices that are in play. One of these is the emphasis on voice classification systems as the best tools for working with changing voices, so this viewpoint is upheld from teacher generation to teacher generation. Few different or new ideas are making it into conversations. I acknowledge that many choral teachers often have limited access to the latest research on the adolescent voice, so new ideas and ways of thinking are, frankly, just not reaching the people who actually work with adolescent singers (unless the teacher happens to take a graduate class that provides access to new research). Some of that responsibility for access falls on larger state and national music education and choral organizations, especially when programming conferences or planning practitioner-focused publications. It is essential that our organizations carefully consider the needs of teachers in today's classrooms and work toward moving the profession forward in thinking and doing, which includes discussion of new research in the field. But before I wander too far off topic, let's go back.

In order to better understand the larger scope of voice classification systems and other foundational ideas in choral music education, it is worth exploring some of the most eminent works in our profession, as well as acknowledging the authors of these works.

1885: EMIL BEHNKE AND LENNOX BROWNE

The first work presented here is not specifically focused on voice classification but *is* completely focused on adolescent vocal development. *The Child's Voice* was the first book of its kind and, as you will see, some of the discussion it contains is still relevant today; other sections are quite progressive, especially for the late 1800s; and other sections of the book expose the limited understanding of the voice during that era. It is a fascinating read.

In the late 1800s Emil Behnke and Lennox Browne attended a lecture given by a leading throat specialist and heard the speaker state that "there is no necessity for boys to abstain from singing during the period of the 'breaking' of their voices" (pp. ix–x). Behnke and Browne were appalled, for they were completely opposed to this perspective and felt that boys should absolutely refrain from singing during voice change. To combat what they heard at the lecture, the two men launched a research study about singing during voice change

> not merely to treat the subject from our own personal experience, both scientific and practical, medical and musical, but to submit a number of questions to those best qualified to judge, thereby giving a value to opinions advanced and treatment recommended far beyond that attaching solely to our own views. (p. x)

Behnke and Browne distributed surveys to students in different music training colleges, voice teachers, and music college officials. They received 200 responses to an eight-item questionnaire and 610 responses to a four-item follow-up questionnaire—a much larger response than anticipated. Their 1885 publication *The Child's Voice* was a compilation of responses to their surveys.

Many different singing-related topics are discussed in *The Child's Voice*, with sections ranging from "Cultivation of the Child's Voice in Relation to Health" and "Singing as a Matter of Musical Education" to "Causes Underlying the Change of Voice in Both Sexes," all supported with commentary from survey participants. There is too much in this book to completely relay here, but I would like to share a few primary topics, the first being *registers* of junior singers. There was no mention of assigning students to a voice part, and explaining what was actually happening in the body was deemed unnecessary; rather, the key was developing awareness of the various vocal registers in the body. The authors wrote,

> Teachers will find, if they have once succeeded in getting a few of their quicker pupils to use the proper registers, that the others will unconsciously adopt the same means of producing their voices; and no difficulty will therefore be experienced on this head. It will not even be necessary to say anything to the children about the registers—much less given them lectures on vocal physiology. (p. 32)

The one mention of singer classification was based on student ability and had nothing to do with vocal range or developmental vocal stage:

> The children should also be more carefully classified with regard to ability than they have been in the former grade, because the quick ones and the slow ones are serious hindrances to each other. The quick pupils are prevented from making progress by the slow ones; and the slow ones are prevented from making progress because they simply follow the lead of the others, and make no independent exertions of their own. But, what is worse, the voices of the quicker pupils are in serious danger of being injured by the terrible strain which is put upon them in their efforts to drag along with them the dead weight of the backwards ones. (pp. 32–33)

I feel compelled to stop for a moment to say that I wish this way of thinking about changing voices was a thing of the long-gone past, but, unfortunately, it is not. Many people still hold this perspective about singers whose voices are changing. There is absolutely no reason why a student should feel bad about the way their voice is progressing through voice change (it certainly is no one's *fault)* and no one benefits from considering changing voices in terms of being quick, slow, or dead weight.

Behnke and Browne reported that some survey respondents "likened the importance of rest during the break of the voice to the necessity for repose of a broken limb" (p. 23), for voice breaking was a very serious problem that required very serious rest:

> All medical authorities agree that at the period of break of the voice there is a state of congestion of the vocal organs, i.e. an increased blood-supply without sufficient allowance of return; and it is strange that any physician should recommend continuance of exercise of vocal function in such a state of things in the case of young boys on the verge of manhood, when his first injunction to an adult patient in similar circumstances would be the observance of complete functional rest. (p. 23)

Although Behnke and Browne preferred to consider voice breaking more as "a sprain of joint or tendon" (p. 23) than as a broken limb, both men tended to agree that complete vocal rest was the best approach to navigating breaking during male voice change. In response to their survey question, "Do you consider it safe for a boy to continue singing while his voice is breaking?" the 190 participants responded (emphasis is in the original in all that follows):

- 2 correspondents say that it *is* safe.
- 11 say it is safe, if the voice be only *moderately used*, and *not strained.*
- 9 say a boy may safely continue to sing if he takes a lower part.
- 3 recommend a lower part *for a time*, and afterwards *perfect rest.*
- 3 deprecate the custom of taking a lower part when the voice breaks.
- 2 comment on the danger of singing too soon after the break, before the voice is settled.
- 11 remark that there is often no *real* break, but only a gradual change.
- 6 give inconclusive replies.
- 6 note certain peculiarities attending the break.
- 158 say that it is *decidedly not* safe for a boy to sing while his voice is breaking. (pp. 64–65)

It is worth seeing some of the direct responses to this question in full, so I selected a few of my favorites from the many that Behnke and Browne provided in *The Child's Voice*:

> MR. EDWIN EDWARDS: If the boy is physically able to sing—i.e. if he can control his voice, and does not by singing bring on coughing or irritation of the throat—he should sing through childhood, youth, and adolescence. (p. 65)

MR. JOHN M. W. YOUNG: I do not think it will injure a boy, or affect his voice afterwards, if he sings *a little and quietly* when his voice begins to change; but on the first indication of a change of voice he should not be allowed to sing any *exercises* or *practise* any more. This has been my plan for many years. (pp. 65–66)

MR. T. ROYLANDS-SMITH: I am of the opinion that youths and young men do not give sufficient time for their manly voices to *settle* before beginning freely to use them. I do not think sufficient time is allowed for the needful rest of the voice during the time the throat is developing; and this is the cause of so many voices of men being of an unmusical character. (p. 67)

DR. BRIDGE: No. I believe that a boy should cease to sing as soon as his voice shows *signs* of breaking. (p. 70)

DR. GARRETT: *Certainly not.* The throat is not in a condition for it in ninety-nine cases out of a hundred. (p. 70)

DR. FREDERICK ILIFFE: *Most unsafe*—a great and almost general mistake. (p. 72)

DR. HORTON ALISON: No. I should think it *certainly useless* and *probably* injurious. (p. 72)

MR. JOHN STORER: No. Decidedly not; *the greatest folly imaginable.* (p. 72)

DR. H. A. HARDING: No. I think it a cruel shame that boys are made to sing at *all* when their voices begin to break; and I attribute the scarcity of real tenors and basses to this practice. (p. 73)

Pause for a moment to consider that if we still followed this line of thinking, there would likely be no boys in our middle or high school choral programs at all. It is remarkably good that our profession (and the medical profession as well, apparently) has moved forward in research and thinking about the larynx since 1885.

Female Voices, Specifically

A striking characteristic of *The Child's Voice* is the amount of focus on the female voice. Some of the discussion is quite insightful, and I am impressed that consideration of female voices was taking place in 1885. That said, much of the commentary reveals wider beliefs about women and their general abilities at the time, so take a bit of what follows with a grain of salt.

Behnke and Browne begin their chapter "Comparison of the Girl's Voice with That of the Woman" by stating, "With regard to girls, there is no actual change of the vocal organ, but simply a development" (p. 47). They go on to explain that male voices are impossible to predict owing to the massive change during puberty, but "a girl singing soprano or contralto will, in the vast majority of cases, preserve the same *class* of voice" (p. 58). In order to further explore this idea, the authors asked several of the leading anatomists and physiologists of the time for a physiological explanation of the matter, and I share some of the doctors' responses here.

> *Dr. James Barr, of Liverpool:* It seems to me that you start with a false premise—"In the case of the boy, the bodily change at puberty is simply one of growth and development." Is there not also an evolution of character both morally and intellectually? Is there not also a varying development in the larynx, vocal cords, &c. which does not occur in the female? You ascribe to the varying length, thickness, &c. of the vocal cords the chief factor in the division of voices. Is it not a fact that many good tenors are rather effeminate and defective in manly traits of character? In females, puberty effects great physical changes in the evolution of sexual functions; but this seems to be chiefly in the direction of child-bearing. There is not the same alteration in character, and what changes there are, are in an opposite direction to those of the male. She becomes more subdued, more modest and retiring, less self assertive and more matronly in her habits." (pp. 58–59)
>
> *Professor Michael Foster, F.R.S., Professor of Physiology in the University of Cambridge:* I would rather say that the bodily change at puberty is in woman [*sic*] more special, and then, the difficulty, if I understand your difficulty aright, will be much less. In the course of the evolution of the sexual characteristics of the adult there has been nothing which has led to any marked change in the voice in woman, but rather the influences have acted to keep it as it was. In man, on the other hand, influences have tended to a marked change in the voice, leading to a great jump at puberty. A somewhat analogous case is the beard; the change in a woman's chin is *nil* at puberty; that in a man's immense!" (p. 59)
>
> *Professor Turner, F.R.S., Professor of Anatomy in the University of Edinburgh, and at the Royal Scottish Academy:* My conception of the difference in voice in the two sexes has been that it was due to the local changes in the larynx itself . . . and not to a generally [*sic*] body change; and which local changes do not occur to anything like the same extent in the female larynx as in the male at the time of puberty. (p. 59)

Behnke and Browne were generally unhappy with the responses because no clear explanation was provided as to why the female larynx did not grow as much as the male larynx during puberty when both sexes experienced significant general body change. They claimed to have examined Charles

Darwin's writings for an answer to their query (which would be accessible because his monumental work had just been published), and on close examination of Darwin's work, wrote:

> Darwin has shown at great length how (1) the use and growth of the vocal organs may have originated during the excitement of love-making; and (2) how, during the struggle of the males for the females among non-polygamous animals, the males made more use of their voices, which consequently developed more completely. They used their voices in love-making, in fighting for the handsomest females, and in the warfare promiscuously carried on during this period. (p. 62)

So there you have it.

Other survey questions by Behnke and Browne included comparisons of the female voice at different stages of life. The inquiry "What is the difference between your woman's voice and your child's voice?" (p. 47) yielded many varied replies. The 219 responses to this specific question emerged as follows:

- 66 know of no difference.
- 13 say that their woman's voice is weaker than their child's voice.
- 56 observe that there is an increase both in strength and volume.
- 30 remark that there is an increase both in strength and compass.
- 17 say that their woman's voice is lower in pitch than their child's voice.
- 16 have changed from soprano to mezzo-soprano.
- 10 have changed from soprano to contralto.
- 5 have changed from mezzo-soprano to soprano.

As with the discussion of male voice change, it is worth examining a few of the full written responses to this question about the difference in the female voice between childhood and adulthood:

> MADAME ANTOINETTE STERLING: In consequence of my exceptionally good constitution, my voice has *always* been—since I can remember—perfectly natural, strong, and healthy. I doubt if there was *much* difference after (say) twelve years of age; but this, I dare say, is exceptional. (p. 48, emphasis in original)
>
> MADAME SEILER: The difference between children's and women's voices, as I experienced in *my own* case, and in the case of all my young pupils, is neither in compass nor in the registers, but in the greater fulness [*sic*] and power of tone, and in a change of *timbre* in the woman's voice. (p. 48)

MR. W. G. MCNAUGHT: A change often obscure and embarrassing does take place in girls' voices, concurrent with their physical development. What to do under these circumstances has always been to me a matter of doubt. (p. 49)

MR. FRANK BRAINE: A girl's voice will *change* many times. I know an instance: viz. at twelve, very high soprano; at sixteen, contralto, until nineteen, when all low notes failed, and the voice settled into clear, powerful mezzo-soprano. (p. 50)

While there is no great finale to *A Child's Voice*, Behnke and Browne made two statements that I hold most dear among all of the writing in their book. The first is the following:

> We are more than ever convinced that, so far as the larynx is concerned, the voice trainer has no business to interfere, or, in other words, that no serious vocal work should be attempted before the voice of the man or of the woman has completely settled. (p. 50)

I agree with this statement and, despite other aspects of the book that I find odd with regard to approaching adolescent voices, I wish that *this* idea was more fully embraced today. In 1885 these researchers came to the conclusion that physiological growth should be allowed to finish before "serious vocal work" was undertaken. My interpretation of Behnke and Browne's term "serious vocal work" includes vocal training limited to one specific voicing or area of the voice, singing demanding vocal repertoire that requires access to extreme areas of the range (high and low), singing for long durations of time without rest, and demanding dynamics (loud and soft). For me, classifying changing voices prior to the conclusion of physiological growth launches adolescent singers into realms of serious vocal work before they are physiologically ready to do so.

The second statement with which I strongly identified came at the end of *A Child's Voice*: "It is a great mistake to think of the voice only as the result of the action of a certain well-defined apparatus. It is, in fact, part and parcel of our entire selves, and affected by all manner of influences entirely" (p. 100). This statement lives deep in the heart of the book you are reading at this very moment. I did not discover Behnke and Browne's work until after I had already decided to write this book and address adolescent voice change in ways not yet overtly addressed in our profession. Perhaps it is a bit of romanticism, but I find it strangely exciting and reassuring that the ideas I hold so dear were also shared by others so long ago, and I feel honored to carry forth this fundamental idea for Behnke and Browne.

The Authors

Emil Behnke died in 1892 at the age of 56. In his obituary, his "highly successful methods" and work to help people with vocal issues were lauded: "Mr. Behnke may be almost said to have created the profession in which he so prominently distinguished himself; a peculiar position, midway between that of a physician and musician, but partaking of the nature of both" (*The Musical Times*, October 1, 1892). His work with the voice led him to become "universally accepted as the leading authority on all matters relating to the voice" (Stiles, 2017, n.p.). Lennox Browne died in 1906 at the age of 65. He was a co-founder of the Central London Throat and Ear Hospital and a highly respected laryngologist. His obituary described him as "of a keen intellect and a masterful force of character" and stated that "he contributed to the literature of his subject with considerable frequency, and, it need hardly be said, was always ready to join in the controversies of the day" (*Journal of Laryngology, Rhinology, and Otology*, December 1902).

Although these men were highly respected for their work with the voice, I am continually struck by the fact that the impetus for their book, *The Child's Voice*, was their belief that people should completely refrain from singing during voice change. This is certainly quite the opposite of the way choral and voice teachers approach the changing voice today. And I am curious as to what degree Behnke and Browne's work and theories influenced music teachers and adolescent singers in the late 1800s and what carries over still today. I also wonder what choral music educators will think about our current considerations of adolescent voices in another 130 years.

1956: DUNCAN MCKENZIE

According to research by music education professor Don L. Collins, Duncan McKenzie taught public school in Montreal and Toronto. He later worked as manager of the music department of Oxford University Press for five years and for Carl Fischer, Inc., for twelve years (both positions in New York). He was also chairman of the Douglass College music department from 1943 to 1952 (Collins, 1999, p. 124). In 1956 McKenzie published *Training the Boy's Changing Voice* to promote the alto-tenor approach for working with adolescent singers. His intention was to counter the "traditional theory" that boys should not sing through voice change and promote the "modern theory" that males should sing throughout voice change, provided a qualified teacher assist with the process. His book was designed to assist musicians within and outside of school systems.

Although McKenzie is known for his alto-tenor plan, he actually did not originate the term. In *Training the Boy's Changing Voice*, McKenzie shared commentary from Eldridge W. Newton, who believed that the term was first used in about 1894: "The term referred to a part which might be sung by a girl alto or by an incipient boy tenor" (p. 21). McKenzie also did some digging and discovered a music textbook from 1885 that he believed to be "the first school text to apply the rudiments of the alto-tenor idea" (p. 22). So whereas McKenzie is often credited with creating the alto-tenor plan, it was actually in existence long before his time. What McKenzie did was tweak this plan so that it could be implemented with adolescent males in American music classrooms. His plan emerged following "years of experience in teaching music in Scotland and Canada, and of observation and consultation with teachers in different parts of America" (p. vii).

McKenzie encouraged choral teachers to monitor the male speaking voice for changes, because a lowering of pitch in the speaking voice indicated that change was taking place in the singing voice, or going to take place soon. Once voice change began, male speaking and singing voices moved from soprano downward through all of the stages during vocal mutation. When the voice reached the "bottom" of the range it eventually rose upward again and settled as a tenor or bass. McKenzie outlined the official vocal stages of the alto-tenor plan as follows:

- Soprano I: unchanged (middle C to G5 [high G])
- Soprano II: Usually still able to sing Soprano I, but the speaking voice has begun to lower. Difficulty singing around a high E or F is a characteristic of a Soprano II. (B3 [right below middle C] to E5 [high E])
- Alto: Once the singer struggles with the higher notes of Soprano II range, he should be moved to Alto. New lower notes are possible. Deeper and full tone is present. (A3 to C5)
- Alto-Tenor: "Alto-tenor" is the term used to describe and classify the boy's voice after it has lowered to the stage when the changed voice begins to develop. "The voice is still alto, but it has lowered to the extent that a boy can sing in the tenor range; the quality, however, has not yet become masculine, that is, either tenor or bass" (p. 19). Fast-transitioning voices are likely destined to be bass; slowly transitioning voices are likely destined to be tenor. Range is typically an octave, but can vary with individual singers. (G3 [below middle C] to G4 [above middle C])
- Tenor: "Since the tenor voice develops so gradually and imperceptibly that it is hard to observe that any change is taking place, it is not possible to say exactly when an alto-tenor becomes tenor" (p. 31). Tenor voices are

"extremely rare" in junior high and "immature" in high school, so repertoire and vocal exercises must be selected carefully. (A singer is classified as a tenor when his range has lowered to C3 [the octave below middle C].)

- Bass: The lowest notes will be sung with the changed voice, not the unchanged. "As long as he sings in a range that is comfortable, there is no harm in his singing the very lowest notes he can produce" (p. 33).

McKenzie promoted preservation of boys' singing voices via a "comfortable range" policy by which an adolescent singer was taught to develop awareness about his voice and sing only within his most comfortable vocal range. McKenzie believed that such practice would greatly benefit adolescent male singers as their voices developed, lowered, and settled.

1965: IRVIN COOPER AND KARL O. KUERSTEINER

In 1965 Irvin Cooper (who was a professor of music education at Florida State University) and Karl O. Kuersteiner (who was dean of the School of Music at Florida State University) published *Teaching Junior High School Music*. This book was intended for general music teachers in that it provided ideas for working with junior high general music students and included activities for singing, music reading, ear training, and listening. The authors wrote their book from a choral perspective in order to help instrumentalists who might end up teaching general music (which could involve the voice) as part of their teaching responsibilities.

One of the most significant aspects of this book was the introduction of their "cambiata plan." The word *cambiata* refers to the first stage of male voice change and was specifically selected to distinguish this classification system from Mackenzie's alto-tenor plan. Cooper and Kuersteiner described the cambiata voice as "truly beautiful" (p. 18) with trademark qualities of being "rich and a trifle *woolly*" (p. 18, emphasis in original). These vocal qualities made the cambiata voice challenging to identify, and teachers often classified this stage of vocal development too low, as a baritone or a bass. To complicate matters, the cambiata voice created an aural illusion that it was one octave lower than it really was, again leading music teachers to classify these voices as baritone or bass, but even tenor lines were too low for cambiata voices to sing.

Five basic types of voices were established by the cambiata plan, presented with the caveat that "it is a gross error to assume that every voice in each category fits precisely the prescribed range boundaries" because both males and females sometimes sing outside the defined ranges (p. 18).

1. Soprano girls (A#3 [below middle C] to F4 [above middle C])
2. Unchanged boys (same range as soprano girls)
3. Cambiata: boys in first change (F3 [below middle C] to C5 [C above middle C])
4. Baritones: boys in second change (A#2 to F4)
5. Bass (rare): boys who have changed (G2 to C4 [middle C])

The authors strongly urged music educators to talk with their students about the different kinds of singing voices, using diagrams to promote understanding. Although they were supportive of singers at all stages of voice change, it was clear from their writing that the cambiata voice was very special to Cooper and Kuersteiner; they cited working with cambiata voices as "the most exhilarating and rewarding experience for the junior high school music teacher" (p. 20).

Female voices. *Teaching Junior High School Music* principally focused on adolescent male voices, but Cooper and Kuersteiner briefly discussed adolescent female voices. They disclosed that girls' voices "are inclined to be thin and sometimes shrill" (p. 17) and, as a result, girls are often categorized as sopranos. But they warned, "A thin voice is not necessarily a high voice; it could be, of course, but this is not the general situation" (p. 18). With regard to female singers with voices of the opposite quality, Cooper and Kuersteiner cautioned that "richer, thicker vocal quality does not necessarily indicate a low voice" (p. 18). While female voices might be characterized as high or low on the basis of temporary adolescent vocal quality, "at this age the vast majority of girls' voices lies [*sic*] within one common range: A#3 (below Middle C)-F5 (high F)" (p. 18).

On a personal note, I greatly respect Cooper and Kuersteiner's comments on the female voice and aspire to see this sentiment embodied more in the choral music education profession. I encourage all to read the previous paragraph again and then once more for good measure.

1965: RICHARD LUCHSINGER AND GODFREY E. ARNOLD

In the same year that Cooper and Kuersteiner published their cambiata plan, two physicians, Richard Luchsinger (associate professor of otolaryngology at the Zurich University Medical School) and Godfrey E. Arnold (associate professor of surgery and director of otolaryngology at the University of Mississippi Medical School), published *Voice-Speech-Language: Clinical Communicology; Its Physiology and Pathology.* The 1965 publication was actually the third iteration of their book. The first edition was published in

German in 1949 as *Lehrbuch der Stimm- und Sprachheilkunde*; the second edition (1959) was twice as long and more complete than the first, and also in German. It was recommended to the authors that they translate their work into English, leading to the third edition in 1965, described in the medical community as "the most authoritative and comprehensive volume on the disorders of the voice and speech" (Luchsinger & Arnold, 1965, p. vi).

Luchsinger and Arnold wrote *Voice-Speech-Language* for medical professionals concerned with disorders of the voice, meaning that the majority of the book lies outside the scope of a discussion of adolescent changing voices. They included detailed discussion of laryngeal anatomy and physiology, as well as the endocrine system (some of which I wove into the introduction and chapter 2 of this book, so I will not go into those particulars again here). It is Luchsinger and Arnold's commentary on female changing voices, however, that has brought this text into choral music education. Their 1965 book has been repeatedly cited in choral education publications referencing the female changing voice to legitimize its existence from a scientific standpoint. I, myself, have repeatedly cited their comment, "It is less known that *girls also undergo vocal mutation*" (1965, p. 134, emphasis in original).

Whereas this 1965 book has been important in establishing the existence of female voice change, it has also been cited as an example of the general perspective that this phenomenon is not a big deal. Luchsinger and Arnold wrote, "As a result of the *different rate of laryngeal growth* in the two sexes, vocal mutation is stormier and more embarrassing in boys than it is in girls" (p. 134, emphasis in original). On a personal note, I have mixed feelings about this publication, because I have appreciated Luchsinger and Arnold's scientific acknowledgment of female voice change. But I am unclear as to why the doctors suddenly crossed the line from reporting the physiological facts to commenting on the assumed emotional well-being of singers with changing voices. It would have been accurate and appropriate to say that, based on the different rates of laryngeal growth, voice change experiences can be different for boys than for girls. However, their published comment reveals author bias about female versus male voice change, leaving me conflicted throughout their scientific discussion of anatomical growth.

1973: FREDERICK J. SWANSON

Frederick J. Swanson was a junior high choral music educator in Moline, Illinois for more than 40 years; he also founded the Moline Boys Choir in

1948, and it still exists today. Swanson originally organized the choir with no plans to use it in his research, but he eventually did so as part of his work. His first book, *Music Teaching in the Junior High and Middle School* (1973), addressed a variety of topics related to working with adolescents in music classes on a broader scale, so it was applicable to choral, band, orchestra, and general music educators working with this population. Of the five sections in the book, the third, "The Boy Challenge," focused on teaching adolescent male singers and, more specifically, how to better meet the needs of boys experiencing voice change. He wrote,

> Since this is a normal event in the stages of growing up, it should not be a traumatic experience, not even a disturbing or thwarting one. Under the tutelage of a knowledgeable teacher, and with full awareness of what is going on, a boy can find this transition fascinating and challenging, and the whole period of change can be an exciting time. (1973, p. 174)

Swanson acknowledged that while male voice change can be challenging and embarrassing and can result in teasing from friends, the entire matter was actually one of grave concern that should receive serious focus in music education. He was frustrated that medical professionals could not contribute more to our understanding of the changing voice and that music educators were not pushing for a deeper physiological understanding of male voice change:

> Many may know that boys' voices change, but few experts can tell why they change or how they change. Even the physiologists and students of adolescent psychology as well as the anatomists become vague and indefinite in their descriptions of the rapid growth of the male larynx in adolescence. So if the beginning teacher decides to go searching for a clear, valid, comprehensive description of how a voice changes as it develops from boyish treble to manly tenor-bass, he may find his search frustrating and unrewarding. (p. 175)

Swanson expressed further irritation because people expressed many opinions in music education, but "objective, reliable descriptions of carefully conducted research are scant. Carefully controlled, reproduceable [*sic*], and measurable studies are scarce" (p. 175). Swanson wrote very passionately about the need for empirical research and seemed to enjoy building suspense in his writing. Therefore, at this point in his chapter I sensed "a huge and steaming bowl of foreshadowing" (*Deadpool 2*, 2018), and for good reason. Ultimately, Swanson revealed data he had collected on voice-change patterns with 82 eighth-grade boys from which he established general groupings for male changing voices (not specific stages of change):

- Treble tones, not yet in voice change.
- Only bass-clef tones, occasionally on the very deep tones of the lower bass clef, with a very restricted range. (Swanson urged teachers to listen carefully to these voices and not dismiss them as deficient; they may be accurately singing "fry tones" or in a "pulse register" an octave below standard bass clef.)
- Literally two voices, one high and one low, quite separate and of distinctly different quality with "an area of silence" between them where no tones could be produced at all. (It is with these voices that Swanson encouraged continued development of the "falsetto tenor" voice to help close the gap between the two voices.)
- An overlap in voices: as the changed voice extended upward and the treble (falsetto) voice extended downward, there were a certain number of pitches that could be sung in either voice. (1973, p. 186; Swanson, 1984, p. 49)

In 1977 Swanson published *The Male Singing Voice Ages Eight to Eighteen*, which focused on teaching the male changing voice. It was informed by large amounts of data that he had collected over the course of thirty years as a private voice teacher, choral teacher, conductor, and clinician, as well as research gathered for his doctoral dissertation. He was very concerned for young boys who sang beautifully and were involved in singing prior to voice change but had no one to help them navigate vocal challenges and frustrations once their voices began to crack; he was troubled by the fact that many of these boys would likely stop singing altogether as a result.

Female voices were barely considered in his conversations, even though Swanson revealed some semblance of awareness of female vocal challenges during adolescence:

> For the moment the girls do not pose so many problems. They have been singing soprano and alto for several years and are probably quite prepared to continue doing so. True, these thirteen-and-fourteen-year-old girls' voices will tend to be colorless, breathy, rather restricted in range. There will be only a few who can be definitely classified as true altos, and there will not be many who can soar above the treble clef with ease as genuine sopranos. But right now they are ready to assume their roles as sopranos and altos; they are not your most urgent problem. (1977, p. 96)

He later wrote in his article "Changing Voices: Don't Leave out the Boys" that "girls' voices change very little in pitch as they move into adulthood, but boys' voices change drastically." (1984, p. 47). These comments suggest to me that Swanson was not ignoring female voices but instead felt that female singers would be fine if not directly attended to; males, however, needed intervention and overt support to continue singing and it was to them that he was fully committed.

Ultimately, Swanson encouraged a positive perspective on the male changing voice and wanted others to embrace the experience of voice change as one of the glass being half full rather than half empty. I leave my discussion on Swanson's work with the following excerpts from his 1977 book that sum up his core belief about the male changing voice:

> The most formidable hazard a boy must overcome in his singing career is vocal mutation. Yet it should not be a hazard, for voice change is a natural phenomenon, a part of growing up that every male child experiences. Hence it is better thought of as a challenge, an intriguing development, an adventure into a newer vocal world. A more mature voice is about to emerge, richer in quality, more powerful in volume, lower in pitch . . . . Every descending tone that is added in the bass clef is an event of interest; a change in quality in the treble range is fascinating; each quirk that develops in the erratic descent is not so much a nuisance as it is a curiosity. (1977, p. 66)
>
> A few dedicated choral directors and junior high school music teachers are not only well-trained musicians, but are also sensitive to the physical and mental workings of that outwardly brash and ebullient, but inwardly sensitive and bewildered human being, the adolescent boy. These rare teachers and directors have made the effort to learn about the phenomenon of voice change and how to exploit it to proper development. They do not dread it as something catastrophic, but look on it as something fascinating. (1977, pp. 66–67)

I find these sentiments to be absolutely lovely and agree wholeheartedly. It is my hope that the larger profession of choral music education, including incoming and future teachers, is provided the opportunity to contemplate Swanson's views about adolescent singers and remember them when working with changing voices.

1977: JOHN COOKSEY

In 1977 John Cooksey began a four-part article series in the *Choral Journal* titled "The Development of a Contemporary, Eclectic Theory for the

Training and Cultivation of the Junior High School Male Changing Voice." In "Part 1: Existing Theories," Cooksey reviewed the work of Irvin Cooper, Frederick Swanson, and Duncan Mackenzie, similarly to my undertaking in this chapter. (Cooksey also disclosed that he was a student of Irvin Cooper, co-author of the cambiata plan. He described Cooper as "a rare, warm, and dynamic teacher, both of college students and junior high school young people" [1977a, p. 7]. I love lineage in the choral profession!) In his article, Cooksey advocated for deeper conversation and further examination of adolescent voice change via peer-reviewed research protocol. He wrote:

> I strongly feel that we, as a profession, must arrive at consensus regarding many of the unresolved questions mentioned above. There must be a full-scale attack on these problems . . . lots of open discussions, local, regional, [and] national symposiums, serious research projects, and continuing dialogue based upon scientific, as well as, empirical evidence. (1977a, p. 6)

Although he did not unveil his Contemporary-Eclectic Theory (C, E Theory) and stages of voice change in Part 1 of this article series, as I read the following passage I was again struck by a sense of foreshadowing.

> We must also look to other sciences such as laryngology, acoustics, speech pathology, and phonetics for ideas. We must dig for ideas in extant research studies, dispassionately discuss the proposals of junior high choral experts, and *freely* share our own opinions. We should not be afraid to hammer out *practical* ways for solving some of the issues raised by the experts. In short, we must develop a contemporary eclectic practical approach for the training and cultivation of the junior high school male changing voice. (1977a, p. 6, emphasis in original)

Cooksey focused on physiological characteristics of puberty in "Part 2: Scientific and Empirical Findings; Some Tentative Solutions" and strongly advocated for increased understanding about male biological development among choral professionals. He also connected voice change with pubertal changes in males, heavily citing works by researchers in medicine and speech pathology. Cooksey identified range, tessitura, and vocal timbre as "the most important ingredients of each stage of vocal development in the adolescent male" (1977b, p. 12) and then (after much anticipation) revealed his five stages of male vocal development. An exciting moment in this article (at least for me) was when Cooksey commented that the range and tessitura guidelines for those five stages "are guidelines and should be interpreted as such" (p. 12). Guidelines! I like to think that Cooksey followed a pirate code of his own.

The Contemporary, Eclectic Theory is unpacked in great detail in "Part III: Developing an Integrated Approach to the Care and Training of the Junior High School Male Changing Voice" (1977c) and applied to practice with singers in "Part IV: Selecting Music for the Junior High School Male Changing Voice" (1978). Elements of each stage will be discussed momentarily, but first, a little pre-clarification. In his original *Choral Journal* articles, Cooksey defined Stage 1 as "Premutation: Boy Soprano Classification" with four stages following. Jumping ahead 15 years, in 1992 Cooksey published the book *Working with the Adolescent Voice* and in 1999 published *Working with Adolescent Voices*. In these books Cooksey's stages were organized in the same manner as in 1977, but the unchanged premutational voice was identified as the precursor to all stages of voice classification and not the starting stage. It is *this* most recent model that I detail below.

- Unchanged voice (premutational): A3 (below middle C) to F5 (high F)
- Stage 1. Midvoice I (early mutation period): soprano characterized by a full, rich voice with much flexibility. Higher pitches are lost. G#3 (below middle C) to C5
- Stage 2. Midvoice II (high mutation period): voice quality is thicker, darker in color, and less resonant. The vocal range is shortened; lower notes may begin to appear and higher notes are less stable. F3 (below middle C) to A4 (above middle C)
- Stage 3. Midvoice IIA (climax of mutation and key transitional period): the peak of voice change, when the voice is most vulnerable to abuse. Sound quality is husky and increased breathiness leads to forcing or pushing the sound; voices are easily damaged during this stage. This is a transitional stage that may pass quickly or last for many months, depending on the person. D3 (below middle C) to F#4 (above middle C)
- Stage 4. New Baritone (stabilizing period; the term *New Voice* is also used to describe this stage): a settling period that occurs around ages 13 to 15. The voice is light and strains to reach high pitches; the bass vocal line is too low for new baritones to sing. "Blank spots" in the vocal range can occur. B2 to D#4 (right above middle C)
- Stage 5. Settling or Developing Baritone (postmutational developmental and re-expansion period; the term *Emerging Adult Voice* is also used to describe this stage): adult-like vocal characteristics are not yet present, but there is an increased range and vocal capability; more consistency in vocal production. The falsetto register is set. G2 (low G) to D4 (right above middle C) (Cooksey, 1999, pp. 12–17)

Cooksey's two books contained much of the same information as did his *Choral Journal* articles from the 1970s; some of the exact wording actually appeared in all publications. It is interesting to note that his 1992 book was titled *Working with the Adolescent Voice* and exclusively focused on male voice change. His 1999 publication, *Working with Adolescent Voices*, contained brief discussion of female changing voices, including mention of Lynne Gackle's (1991) stages of the female changing voice (you will read about these shortly). Though he acknowledged Gackle's work, Cooksey remained steadfast in his advocacy for empirical research, stating, "While the stages have not been scientifically tested, they should be recognized as a significant step in recognizing and dealing with specific vocal problems of adolescent female singers" (1999, p. 8).

Cooksey retired from formal teaching and conducting in 2006. He passed away in 2012 at the age of 70 after a five-year battle with cancer. One obituary noted:

> Cooksey's passion for choral music and his unflinching desire for his students to excel left a lasting memory for all, not only those who became choir teachers, but for thousands of others who continue to love, listen and sing choral music. (*Deseret News*, November 3, 2012)

I really enjoyed writing this chapter and digging into the works of choral experts whom I have heard about for decades. Sadly, I have come to realize in this process that many of the nuances of the significant work these people accomplished during their careers have, over time, faded away. What we know of them and their work (and what we continually discuss) are small and simplistic pieces of the bigger pictures. For example, I have heard about Cooksey's C, E Theory since my undergraduate days, but my understanding for years was simply that Cooksey established stages of male voice change. Yes, Cooksey's system has remained in the forefront of choral music education as *the* classification system to reference for the adolescent male changing voice, but what is not emphasized about him is his strong advocacy for *research* and *scientific grounding* of findings. Right from the beginning of his first article in 1977, Cooksey made it very clear that evidence mattered and that "the profession needs some scientific and empirical answers" (1977b, p. 5). Nor did I know that he was a student of Irvin Cooper, who himself made significant contributions to the profession. And so forth. All of this is to say that it is worth the time to go to the primary sources of information every once in a while to truly understand how a theory or method or belief system began. If we, as choral educators, continue to only know what we know based on a chain of summaries in other people's work, we lose important details of the primary source and begin to formulate a simulacrum of understanding of their work instead of a true understanding of the vision and purpose behind it.

1991: LYNNE GACKLE

Lynne Gackle wrote "The Adolescent Female Voice: Characteristics of Change and Stages of Development," published in the *Choral Journal* in 1991. This article was the first of its kind, for no one had yet determined stages of vocal development for adolescent female singers; the only stages in use focused on the male changing voice. Right from the start of her article, it was clear that Gackle cared deeply about healthy vocal development of adolescent singers, regardless of sex. Before discussing the stages of girls' vocal development, she implored choral teachers to have knowledge of five key topics:

1. An understanding of how the adolescent voice matures in order to give proper guidance to the development of voice skills and the selection of music.
2. An understanding of the potentials, limitations, characteristics, and unique qualities that may be encountered in individual adolescent voices.
3. A working knowledge of ways to assess the present vocal and musical abilities of each young singer, and ways to help them develop healthy, efficient personal voice skills for self-expression in speaking and singing.
4. A working knowledge of how to choose music that is within the physiological capabilities of young changing voices, and how to appropriately assign vocal parts so that vocal skills are facilitated rather than impeded.
5. The ability to aurally recognize when adolescent voices are speaking and singing efficiently and healthily within their developmental capabilities, or are speaking and singing inefficiently and unhealthily. (Gackle, 1991, p. 17)

As Gackle segued to the female changing voice, she acknowledged a lack of publications and information about the subject, citing as a possible reason that the phenomenon was much more noticeable in males than in females. She stated that "through the years, the assumption has been accepted that the female voice does not really *change*, but instead merely *develops* during the adolescent period" (p. 18, emphasis in original), citing the respected choral director Father William Finn (1939), who wrote in

The Art of the Choral Conductor, "The girl's nature will develop rather than undergo change, and her throat will attest this fact by merely growing, escaping the anatomical readjustments of her brother" (p. 121).

Through "a synthesis of current professional opinion as a review of research regarding the characteristics of the female changing voice" (p. 18), Gackle proposed the following as characterizations of female voice change. (Notice that this is what Cooksey (1999) was referencing when he commented that Gackle's work had not been scientifically tested):

- Insecurity of pitch
- Development of noticeable register breaks (quality changes)
- Increased huskiness in the voice
- Decreased and inconsistent range capabilities (tessitura tends to fluctuate)
- Voice cracking
- Hoarseness
- Generally uncomfortable singing or difficulty in phonation
- Singing heavy tones
- Feelings of heavy, breathy, or rough tone and/or colorless tone
- Breathy, thin quality to the voice
- Lowering of speaking fundamental frequency (1991, pp. 18–21)

Also in this 1991 publication, Gackle first introduced the idea of female voice change as shades of change:

> Perceptually, female voice change can best be described as *shades of change*. If the color blue is suggested, the mind may conjure many different shades of blue—from azure to royal or navy blue—with many colors represented in between. In many ways, color association is an appropriate way to understanding the development of the female voice. The overall color is that of a treble sound—it does not change. However, in terms of *richness, depth*, and *warmth*, the quality changes noticeably, and those stages of change can readily be identified by a trained listener. (Gackle, 1991, p. 21, emphasis in original)

In 2006 Gackle reconceptualized her description, changing the word *stages* to *phases* because of "the *gradual* nature of the changing process over time" (p. 32, emphasis in original). In her 2011 book (which will be explored shortly), she included male voices in the analogy as well:

> Changes of Color vs. Shades of Change: When comparing the voices of boys and girls, it is notable that, at ages six, seven, and eight, their voices seem similar

in tone, range, and color. In fact, please allow me to make a quantum leap and apply a visual analogy to this aural phenomenon. Let's ascribe the color azure (light blue) to both voices as a way to visually characterize their color. As the boy's voice approaches mutation, there is a brilliance in the maturing male soprano which we could liken to a deeper shade of blue. Clarity of tone and brilliance in certain ranges seem effortless in the young boy's voice especially just prior to the beginning of voice mutation.

. . . Thus, as the boy's voice changes the "octave phenomenon" becomes apparent as the voice will lower approximately an octave in an adult male voice. As this happens, the original blue color of the treble voice doesn't change in shade so much as it changes in color. The voice moves through many different colors in the color spectrum—red, green perhaps, etc.

By contrast, as the girl's voice begins to change, the characteristic brilliance of a treble tone is not as pronounced as it is in the boy's voice. . . . As the female voice develops, the azure blue vocal color changes to a deeper blue, to a royal blue, to a navy blue—still a treble voice, still blue, but a different shade of blue. (2011, pp. 13–14)

Gackle determined her classifications of female vocal development based on "10 years of observation with female adolescent voices." She warned that, because every voice is unique, "chronological ages are given as general guides and are not to be used as definitive rules of classification" (1991, p. 21). (This statement again brings to mind the pirate code and my great desire to see classification systems used as supportive tools or guides and not hard-and-fast rules.) Using criteria of mean speaking pitch, vocal range or tessitura, register breaks, and voice quality, Gackle identified the four classifications of female voice change as follows:

- Stage I (prepubertal) typically includes females aged eight to ten. The mean speaking pitch is C4 (middle C) or D4. The vocal range is B-flat3 (below middle C) to F5. Characteristics of a Stage I voice are a light, flute-like sound with no obvious register breaks. The voice is flexible and has a soprano quality similar to that of unchanged male voices at the same age.
- Stage IIA (pubescent or pre-menarcheal) typically includes females aged 11 to 12 and is the first stage of vocal maturity. It is at this time that females also experience the first stages of physical maturity. The mean speaking pitch is B3 to C#4 and the vocal range is A3 to G5. Characteristics of this stage are breathiness in the voice and a loss of pitches in the lower singing range. Singing becomes difficult and uncomfortable; females are not capable of singing loudly. Female head-voice tone is much breathier than the fuller chest-voice tone.

- Stage IIB (pubertal or post-menarcheal) typically includes females aged 12 to 14 and is the peak stage of vocal mutation. The mean speaking pitch is A3 to C#4 and the vocal range is A3 to F5. Stage IIB is the most critical and frustrating time for female singers. Range can be limited upward or downward; register breaks and cracking voices make singing very difficult and uncomfortable. Vocal characteristics during this stage often lead female singers to believe they are chronically sick. It is during this vocal stage that female singers are inappropriately categorized as altos, so it is of utmost importance that singers keep vocalizing their entire range as best they can.
- Stage III (young adult or post-menarcheal) typically includes females ages 14 to 17. The mean speaking pitch is G#3 to B3 (below middle C) and the vocal range is A3 to A5. The range has increased upward at this stage, and there is a consistency in the voice when switching between registers. Breathiness is reduced, vibrato naturally appears, and vocal tone is deeper and richer. Singers find phonation to be much easier; volume, resonance, and vocal agility increase. (1991, pp. 22–23; 2011, pp. 21–24)

Ophelia. In 2006 Gackle published the article "Finding Ophelia's Voice: The Female Voice During Adolescence" in the *Choral Journal.* She summarized literature published between 1949 and 2000 concerning voice care, human development, and the female voice during adolescence and puberty; she also provided details about classifying adolescent female singers. At the conclusion of the article Gackle introduced her association of such singers with Shakespeare's Ophelia:

> This reference to Ophelia, the tragic young character in Shakespeare's *Hamlet*, is very appropriate in terms of female adolescence. Ophelia's life demonstrates the destructive forces that affect young women during adolescence. As a girl, Shakespeare's Ophelia is a typical happy-go-lucky child, but in adolescence, she loses herself. Torn between pleasing those around her (her value being determined by the approval of others much like girls today value themselves through peer approval and society), she is torn apart and loses her life as she desperately seeks to please others. (Gackle, 2006, pp. 34–35)

Gackle left readers with the sense that a bigger conversation was brewing (more foreshadowing!) as her focus in the article shifted from classification of female voices to helping female singers "navigate not only the changes of the voice, but also, the often-harsh realities of adolescence" (2006,

p. 35). She closed the article with a question—"Could it be that by finding Ophelia's voice, we open Ophelia's heart?" (p. 35)—which was a beautiful way to leave this particular paper and go forth to expand the ideas fully in a book.

The book *Finding Ophelia's Voice, Opening Ophelia's Heart* (2011) significantly magnified concepts touched on in Gackle's 1991 and 2006 articles, including detailed diagrams of laryngeal anatomy, strategies, vocal technique exercises, musical considerations, and literature preparation and rehearsal tips for working with adolescent female voices. The final two chapters, "Opening Ophelia's Heart" and "Ophelia Speaks," swirled around notions of self-concept, self-identity, and self-efficacy in connection with developing female voices. The latter chapter relayed direct quotations from female singers (ranging in age from 11 to 36) about their voices, adolescent voice change, and involvement with singing in their lives. Of the many compelling comments, here are a few from adult female interviewees:

BETH H.: In junior high, I remember experiencing breathiness in my voice. It was scary because I felt like it may not come back to its former level of clarity and beauty. I was losing part of myself. As I continued attending choir rehearsals and giving my all, I noticed my voice cracking at least once in every single practice. I didn't think I was straining or doing anything wrong, but I felt helpless to stop. (I understood and felt much better when our choir attended a college lecture and I heard several friends' voices going through similar vocal changes.) (p. 125)

KATRINA M.: During high school voice lessons, I recall my voice becoming "bigger." I struggled with this, because I'd been singing so long and suddenly it felt different. When I felt like I had mastered my new voice, and was able to sing with a consistent tone throughout my range, I felt very empowered as a singer! (p. 126)

MEGAN G.: There was a time when I couldn't sing certain notes when I shifted something in my singing mechanism. . . . I felt slightly unconfident and sad when I couldn't sing those notes. (p. 127)

MANDY T.: I remember when I could not sing as high, purely, and freely as I had in the past. There was hesitation because I knew my voice wouldn't allow me. I felt a slight "musical identity" crisis because I could no longer produce those soaring notes I once could; somehow like I wasn't good enough anymore. (p. 127)

Adolescent female interviewees shared captivating comments about vocal challenges and voice change:

> I wish I could sing as high as I once could, and I hate how at moments my voice sounds breathy. It made me feel like, "Oh my gosh, what's going on?" It scared me a little.
>
> It made me feel self-conscious because I don't know if I sound bad.
>
> It makes me notice how odd and interesting voices are. I sometimes am afraid I am getting worse, though.
>
> These changes don't make me feel any different.
>
> These changes are going to happen so I'm okay with them.
>
> It makes me feel like I don't want to sing out . . . just stand there moving my mouth.
>
> Sad, mad, and a failure.
>
> Well, I think my voice may be evolving. It might be because of puberty, I guess . . . ?
>
> It makes me happy because I know my voice is changing and I am growing up. (Gackle, 2011, pp. 143–144)

I started teaching choir in 1998, and from the get-go I was aware of Lynne Gackle as someone who is upheld with great respect in the choral profession. I am deeply appreciative not only of her work to bring attention to the female changing voice but also of her work to empower *all* female voices. She is a remarkable person and musician, and choral music education is stronger because of her.

DIGEST

The choral education profession has a long history, much more than can be fully explored here. Through linear examination of some of the most influential contributors to our understandings of adolescent voice change, we can see how ideas were fostered, how existing frameworks influenced the creation of new frameworks, and how deep dedication to certain ideas has persisted over the years. Longitudinal awareness is important in a field like choral music, especially as we get older while our classes stay the same age. We benefit from understanding the larger picture.

However, I have some concerns that go back to the beginning of the chapter. I worry that new research is not being conducted and new ways of thinking about voice change or reexaminations of existing ideas about it are not being explored in the wider choral profession. I then worry that, instead of being inspired by new ways to consider adolescent voice change resulting from new explorations via peer-reviewed research protocols, the same perceptions of the voice change experience from the last 130 years will continue to be transferred, unchanged or unchallenged, from generation to generation of choral teachers. I worry that adolescents will stop singing because they need empowerment, acknowledgment, and care in more ways than ever before and if we, as choral educators do not respond to the greater needs of adolescents during voice change, then they will stop singing and we will go extinct. Yes, go ahead and sense foreshadowing.

I encourage all choral teachers to evade complacency and continue exploring new ideas put forth in choral music education, voice and hearing science, adolescent psychology, and so forth. You don't have to like the new ideas, but when you compare new ideas against your current practice, you will either more solidly ground yourself in your beliefs or you will be challenged and inspired to consider new methods moving forward. All experiences are learning experiences, especially if we pause and examine how we react to them. The more we understand about the bigger picture of adolescent voice change, the better we can meet the multifaceted needs of our students, female and male. To get you started on this process, chapter 6 provides some alternative considerations of the adolescent changing voice.

CHAPTER 6

Emerging Considerations

The optimist sees the donut, the pessimist sees the hole.

Oscar Wilde

My own experiences as a singer have planted me firmly in the camp of avoiding permanent classification of young and changing voices by voice part. I have been singing forever and started playing the piano in third grade, so I have always had a good, musical ear. In sixth grade I became the anchor for the alto section because I could hear and hold the harmony parts. I recognize now that my voice was changing in middle school because singing in my chest voice was easy (especially in a belty fashion) but singing anything moderately high was challenging. In seventh and eighth grades my choir teacher kept me in the alto section because, again, I had a good ear and could hold the alto part; we also needed strength on the alto part and I was able and willing to provide that. There is a video of my choir singing "This Little Light of Mine" when I was in seventh grade and, let me tell you, I *dominated* that harmony section, so much so that you can hardly hear anyone besides me. Apparently, I did not grasp the concept of blend or balance at the time, but I sure had a lot of fun belting out that part! I exuded confidence because singing low was easy for me; singing high was terrifying because my high voice was thin and unpredictable and embarrassing.

I distinctly remember a joint venture that involved my middle school choir integrating itself with one of the high school choirs on the choral risers. I was placed in the alto section and one of the high school singers said to her choir director in a snarky tone, "She's an alto?" and the high school director responded, "*Yes*. And a very good one." I was shocked that the high school director knew who I was and saw me as a strong alto singer. That was it: identity as an alto *sealed*. I sang second alto throughout high school and college, as an adult in a "professional amateur" choir, and throughout graduate school.

It wasn't that I did not want to sing high voice parts during all those years. I was terrified of the top part of my voice because I never used it, and no one had ever put me on anything else during my nonstop years in choir. It was not even suggested to me as an option: "Hey, Bridget, you've never sung second soprano before. Want to give it a shot?" Because I did not know what to do with my upper range, I never came forward on my own to volunteer to sing a higher voice part because I was terrified of embarrassing myself. My undergraduate voice teacher was not supportive, and because I was a music education major and not a vocal performance major, she (a former professional opera singer) did not have much of an opinion of me and my singing abilities. My fear of singing high only frustrated her, which did not help me overcome any hurdles. The older I became, the less I used my upper range, and the more nervous I was to sing high in front of others, even as an adult. "You want me to sing in your wedding? Sure! Happy to! Give me the absolute lowest arrangement of every song that you want and you've got a deal!" The story has a happy ending, though: during my doctoral program I took a semester's worth of voice lessons for fun and worked with Anne Nispel at Michigan State University. It was *life changing.* Professor Nispel took the time to understand my voice, instill confidence in me, and help me come to terms with the fact that my upper voice is actually pretty nice. Finally, at the age of 30-something, I found my whole voice.

Again, *I am not anti-classification* but I worry about labeling young voices when they are not ready to be officially labeled, whether the student be a treble or a bass. As discussed in chapter 2, singing voices continue to develop well into the twenties and thirties. How then, can a 12-year-old be told that he is a tenor or bass or that she is an alto or soprano when the voice has 15–20 more years of vocal development ahead? If we think of it in regard to sports, it would be ludicrous to tell a 12-year-old, "Congratulations! You are a second baseman for the rest of your life!" or "Guess what? You are a point guard for the rest of your life!" because that person has not finished physically growing yet. Then why do we, as choral educators, do this with changing voices?

As continuation of the discussion in chapter 5, this chapter involves emerging considerations of adolescent voice change beyond classification systems to provide new food for thought about working with the adolescent changing voice. Before continuing, I want to say that I do understand that many choral educators are very mindful of their students' voices and work hard to help them in the best ways possible; I have met many of you and applaud all of your efforts! I encourage you to share your vision and practices with others, especially new music educators, to initiate new ripple effects in the profession to support and honor all that adolescent voice change encompasses for female and male singers.

THE FEMALE VOICE

While we want to attend to all of our adolescent singers during voice change, I desire to bring some new attention to female voice change via this book to boost considerations of females in choir. With that goal in mind, this section specifically addresses female singers.

The Adolescent Alto

There is a phenomenon in choral education referred to as the "adolescent alto," which involves classifying adolescent female voices based on vocal quality during voice change. (See Cooper and Kuersteiner [1965] in chapter 5 as an example.) As a result, too many female adolescent singers begin to think, "I can't sing ______ because I'm a ______" before physical growth is complete. This mainly happens to singers who temporarily lose their upper range during voice change and are, therefore, classified as altos and kept on alto for a long while. Over time, they gain confidence on the low voice part and, because they are not gaining experience with the other end of their singing range, assume that they are only good at singing low. In my teaching career, I have also encountered the "adolescent soprano," who is the flipped version of what was just described: this student thinks she can only sing high and cannot sing low. I have also worked with several men who have experienced this phenomenon as an "adolescent tenor" or "adolescent bass." Locking onto a specific identity at a young age—whether that be alto, soprano, tenor, bass, or otherwise—limits full vocal and musical potential for singers with changing voices. The younger the singers, the more rooted they can become in such an identity and the less willing (and more scared) they can be to attempt singing outside that identity. This was my experience, as described above; I was a classic case of an adolescent alto.

Collegiate choral conductor Robert L. Harris published the article "The Young Female Voice and Alto" in *Choral Journal* in 1987. This was a forward-thinking article about the adolescent female voice printed prior to the publication of Gackle's full set of female stages of voice change. Harris started out with a bang:

> A surprisingly large number of choral conductors working with immature female voices are willingly, if perhaps unknowingly, abusing the voices of a shockingly large number of their singers. I would suggest that the majority of the young girls who are singing alto parts in elementary, junior high, and even high school choruses are developing vocal habits that will drastically impeded their future vocal development, and in some cases, even sustain vocal damage. Harsh words? Read on! (Harris, 1987, p. 21)

They are not harsh from my perspective. I think Harris is spot on and I am delighted by his honesty. He went on to say that female voices should not be categorized, especially as an alto or mezzo-soprano, at a young age; that many singers are placed on lower choral parts for reasons other than their vocal range; and that staying in the same vocal place is detrimental to vocal development, especially if that place is chest voice. Here's a bit more detail about these main points from his article:

> First, the true contralto is probably the rarest voice type of all. A Marian Anderson or a Kathleen Ferrier is not likely to come through the door of your rehearsal room next semester. Even a mature mezzo-soprano is not likely to be encouraged by her voice teacher to constantly sing in her lower octave and never in her upper head voice. Why then, should we expect a thirteen year old voice to thrive and prosper in the same register? There are very few young singers who belong in the alto section for reasons of vocal range and quality alone, which brings us to the second point.
>
> Who are the leaders of the typical middle school alto section? Is the first qualification a strong, rich, low register? All too often the alto is the one who has the (mis)fortune to have had a few piano lessons, or the natural aptitude to hang on to the harmony part, resisting the temptation to succumb to "melody-itis." They are put there for *non-vocal*, musical reasons. The problem is that girls become convinced, after a couple of years of belting out alto parts, that they ARE altos. Worse, they develop such a habit of singing everything in chest voice that it is extremely difficult to break the old vocal pattern, which brings us to point three.
>
> After the vocal pattern has been established it is very difficult for most singers to get out of the habit of carrying alto chest voice up into their true soprano middle voice, and in many cases, virtually impossible to get up into top head voice without a lot of patient studio training. To put it simply, even though there may not be pathological damage done to the instrument itself, there is still

> substantial vocal-*technical* damage that can be almost as lethal in the long run. At best the singer is in for a frustrating period of adjustment that is not necessary. (Harris, 1987, pp. 2122, emphasis in original)

To assist with ending the practice of generating the adolescent alto (or soprano, tenor, bass), many considerations for working with changing voices are provided at the end of the chapter.

New Qualitative Inquiry

I was invited to write the chapter "Qualitative Choral Music Research" for *The Oxford Handbook of Qualitative Research in American Music Education* (2014), which involved tracking down the choral-focused peer-reviewed qualitative research published in the United States since qualitative research began. It was an interesting project and also quite insightful. At the conclusion of my chapter I wrote,

> The perspectives of adolescent male singers are strongly represented in published research; however, no qualitative research specifically focused on female adolescent choir students, even with urging from researchers such as O'Toole (1994, 2000, 2005). In fact, authors of studies on adolescent male choral students often suggested future research with adolescent female choristers, but nothing has yet been completed and published. (Sweet, 2014, p. 444)

After writing the book chapter, I was incredibly motivated to officially document adolescent female voice change via the process of music education research protocol and peer review. I applied for a Creative Research Award grant at the University of Illinois and began my new line of qualitative inquiry.

A Phenomenological Investigation. My first qualitative study of female voice change was "The Adolescent Female Changing Voice: A Phenomenological Investigation" (Sweet, 2015). I followed phenomenological protocol for this study because it "operates with the assumption that there is an essence to an experience that is shared with others who have also had that experience" (Mariall & Rossman, 2011, p. 20). I studied 14 female choral students in grades 6–12 (two per grade level) across an academic school year at the Durham School of the Arts in Durham, North Carolina. The choral directors, Amy Davis and Sean Grier, identified female students who demonstrated a variety of degrees of voice change characteristics (from vocal breathiness to limited vocal range) and students who were believed "to have something to say" (Sweet, 2015, p. 77). I interviewed each student at three different points during the school year (fall, winter, and spring) and each student also responded to writing prompts on three occasions.

As I describe findings from this study, I reiterate that I launched this research in order to document adolescent female voice change using official protocol. So while some of the findings may seem commonsensical, they have now been officially acknowledged through peer-reviewed qualitative research process, beyond anecdotal evidence. I think John Cooksey would be pleased.

The 14 female participants experienced vocal challenges, including a complete lack of phonation in certain areas of vocal range, excessive breathiness of tone, vocal unpredictability, a lack of strength or endurance when singing, limited vocal range, and difficulties transitioning across registers. These challenges were identical to those documented for adolescent male singers by Kennedy (2004) and Killian (1997). I also found that the participants self-identified with a specific voice part or range prior to the conclusion of laryngeal growth.

Words such as *frustration, embarrassment*, and *pride* illustrated emotions that the female participants encountered during their voice change experiences, the same descriptive words used by their male counterparts (Kennedy, 2004; Killian, 1997). Several females felt alone during vocal challenges, even when singing with others; similar feelings of isolation were reported during male voice change by Elorriaga (2011) and Freer (2006, 2009). In addition, female students felt empowered when their voices responded consistently, especially after warm-ups and longer periods of vocalization; this finding was akin to findings regarding male singers who also reported feeling empowered in similar singing situations (Elorriaga, 2011; Freer, 2009; Kennedy, 2002).

Phenomenological research concludes with an "essence" of a specific phenomenon; in this case it is the shared experience of adolescent female voice change. I think of the essence as a wine reduction or the cooking down of all the findings into a core takeaway. In this study, the essence of the experience of female voice change was that "vulnerability and fear of embarrassment determined all use of the singing voice, resulting in risk assessment for each singing situation and setting" (Sweet, 2015, p. 84). It is important to remember that this study took place in a *school of the arts*, where there is an implied understanding that students will be involved in artistic activities. If fear and vulnerability are determining female students' use of their voice in an arts setting, how are female singers feeling and operating in non-arts settings? That question is definitely something to investigate further.

A main implication from this research is that it provided substantiation that regardless of the severity of voice change, female singers struggle with physical and emotional challenges similar to those of males during adolescent voice change. Therefore:

> There should not be a severity threshold that limits or withholds assistance from female adolescent singers, especially with knowledge that they are self-deprecating or feel "humiliated" from physiological occurrences out of their control. To disregard such challenges and struggles, we discount the experiences of our changing-voice female singers and potentially expose them to the same psychological and emotional risks with which adolescent male singers have struggled (Freer, 2006, 2009, 2010; Kennedy, 2002; Killian, 1999)." (Sweet, 2015, p. 85)

I am reminded of my children. I have a son and a daughter, and if they decide to participate in choir someday, I want to know that both of their voices will be attended to, regardless of severity of voice change. That my son's voice and any vocal challenges will not be given priority over my daughter's because he is a boy and she is a girl.

A Constructionist Examination. While digging into published research for my 2015 study, I came across previous studies for which adult males reflected on their adolescent voice change. I could not find a comparable peer-reviewed empirical qualitative study that examined female voice change in that way, so I launched "Voice Change and Singing Experiences of Adolescent Females" (Sweet, 2018). Instead of following phenomenological protocol, this study followed a constructionist framework. Patton (2015) wrote that "a constructionist would seek to capture diverse understandings and multiple realities about people's definitions and experiences of the situation. A singular or universal explanation would not be sought" (p. 122). My goal was "not to seek a universal explanation but to document multiple understandings and personal realities about experiences surrounding adolescent female voice change" (Sweet, 2018, p. 5).

I interviewed 17 college women at a large midwestern university (not the University of Illinois) to understand how adolescent female voice change had impacted their singing experiences since the age of 11. The findings are especially poignant for the choral music education profession, and some will be mentioned here; see the full article for all findings and supporting discussion.

Vocal challenges during voice change manifested significantly in female participants' emotional and psychological responses to singing experiences, and often resulted in negative self-perspectives and insecurities about their singing ability as adults. Challenges cited included phonation issues (cracking voice, breaks, weakness, unpredictability), difficulty with volume control and blending with others, lack of flexibility, loss of color in the voice, and much tension in their instrument. (So, again, I was officially documenting female vocal challenges via research protocol.) One participant, Caroline, shared, "I think it was in that period from either 11 or 12 to maybe 15 or 16 that I really felt I couldn't sing" (p. 8). Many of the participants remembered having to force or push their voices to produce notes during voice change as a result of vocal challenges. Because of all of their vocal struggles, these women experienced significant stress related to their singing voice, and many were horribly mean to themselves:

> I would just beat myself up and continually tell myself that if my voice wasn't perfect on one day and didn't do exactly what I wanted it to do, then I was, therefore, a terrible musician or a terrible person or why wasn't I good enough? (Mary Ann, p. 8)

Unfortunately, participants' voice change memories and recalled experiences involved negative emotions much more than positive, including sadness, fear, self-doubt, and insecurity. They admitted struggles with confidence and insecurity as adult singers because singing high or singing low was so challenging as adolescents; they carried residue of their voice change experiences with them.

Another finding raised concerns about teacher influence and ensemble-centric considerations, for many of the participants' choral teachers used female singers as mechanisms for maintaining the larger choir's well-being and placed the needs of the choir above the needs of individuals. In addition, many participants felt that being assigned to sing a specific voice part in middle or early high school, and rarely singing notes outside that voice part (sometimes for all of their involvement in choir), severely limited their vocal development and singing potential. One reported,

> I think with boys in choir it's so accepted that, "Oh you're a tenor now but in two years you'll be a bass" where with girls it's more like, "Oh this is what you are when you're five; this is what you are forever." (Avery, p. 10)

The female participants trusted their choral teachers, but my study revealed that many of them sacrificed their own vocal health or development rather than make a request to sing a different part or not sing a certain part (even if they were in physical pain as a result) because they did not want to "hurt" the overall choir or go against the choir teacher. This research stressed the importance of students' not losing their figurative voice during navigation of their literal voice and also stressed the importance of encouraging female singers' self-advocacy. In fact, participants often discussed self-advocacy during their interview and, if it were possible to go back in time, would tell their adolescent selves to speak up and advocate for what they needed or wanted for their voices—especially if something was uncomfortable or painful to sing. One told me,

> I'd definitely go back to my high school self and tell her to advocate more for what's appropriate. If you're not feeling like you can sing it, don't be the Soprano I diva and be like, "*Oh yeah!* I'm singing the B-flat!" Tell someone that doesn't feel right. (Ashley, p. 11)

According to the experiences of these participants, many vocal challenges and needs of adolescent female singers are not acknowledged or met in choir, especially for those experiencing voice change.

One more note from this study: As choral educators, it is important for our female singers to understand that vocal development is not something that is finished by the end of high school. Several of the undergraduate participants believed that their best singing years were now behind them. There was no room for the following exchange in my final published research paper, so this comes from an interview transcript; I am fascinated by it.

> ERIN: I'm happy with how my voice is now, but it could have been so much better. I wish I would have gotten more serious with it, because looking back it was like I had *potential*, like I had it and now I'm here. . . . I mean it all ended up well, but I could be doing so many different things in my life. Like, I could be really serious into music and I could stand at a different point of my life now.
>
> BRIDGET: Your life is not over, though.
>
> ERIN: Yeah, I know.
>
> BRIDGET: You have a lot of life left to live. How old are you?
>
> ERIN: Seventeen.

Conversely, two of the older participants were graduate students in their early and mid-30s, and these women recognized that their vocal challenges had resolved with age. For example, Renee commented:

> I would say that only in the last two years of my life, now I'm thirty-six, things have actually started to come together for me and I feel like the breath is connected to resonant space and I can hit all the high notes and all the muscles are working together. (p. 10)

If only the seventeen-year old who made the preceding comment realized that she had *at least* 20 more years of vocal development ahead, if she wanted it. Somewhere along the line, however, she did not get that message.

Female Vocal Identity. Conducting research is fun, especially because of all the new questions raised in the process. During my 2018 study with the college women, hints of singer identity development poked up occasionally, but not enough to declare it a finding. In conversations with my dear friend and choral music education colleague at Temple University, Elizabeth Cassidy Parker, it was decided that a study exploring female vocal identity was warranted. Together we launched the study "Female Vocal Identity: A Phenomenology" (Sweet & Parker, 2018).

The purpose of our research was to investigate influences on female singers' vocal identity development and how those influences shaped participants' futures as musicians and music educators. As indicated by the title, this was a phenomenological study. We interviewed 39 students from freshman year through graduate school at two large universities in the United States (one in the Midwest, one in the Northeast) enrolled in vocal music education or vocal performance programs. I am going to share the essence before embarking on details of our findings (remember, the essence is like a wine reduction): Intrapersonal and interpersonal interactions, both past and present, determined female vocal musicians' perceptions of their voice and influenced their ever-evolving relationship with their instrument (Sweet & Parker, 2018, p. 14). *Intrapersonal* interactions occurred within the self or within one's mind, while *interpersonal* interactions indicated relationships and communication between people. As with the studies reviewed above, I will share some of the findings; the remaining discoveries can be gleaned from the full published report.

Participants identified choral and voice teachers as powerful influences in labeling and reinforcing their emerging vocal identities. Choral teachers were consistently held in high esteem, and the female participants described how choral teachers generally enhanced their enjoyment of involvement with the choir. However, because choir teachers' focus remained on the ensemble rather than on individual singers, they felt that their voice part was related to, and a result of, the needs of the whole choir and the way their individual voices contributed to it. As such, participants often said that they could not or should not speak up about their assigned voice part, as they feared responsibility for diminishing the larger choir. (Note: This finding comes from a new study with new participants and new data, yet notice the similarity with the findings of my 2018 solo study.)

For many of the women we interviewed, voice classification was solidified at a young age and had become a permanent facet of their vocal identity. It was an important source of their individuality. As one told us,

> Moving into high school I didn't have any other musical experiences outside of being an alto, so I consistently told various choir directors that I was an alto, and after they heard my chest voice they agreed. I took so much pride in the fact that I was an alto. There was something special about not being a girly soprano and actually having to learn harmonies. (Abbey, in Sweet & Parker, 2018, p. 10)

That said, participants' voice classification sometimes clashed with their self-perceptions. This resulted in internal conflict that manifested in a fear of singing, especially as an adult, and a negative opinion of their singing abilities in one vocal range or another. One singer stated,

> My "voice-part conflict" has profoundly impacted my voice and qualities as a musician. Because I spent so long as an alto developing my lower voice, I have incredible anxiety when I'm asked to sing a soprano solo in front of others; singing in my voice studio is an incredible challenge for me. Because I am not entirely confident with my label as a soprano, this lack of confidence really channels itself into my performances. I have also found that through my study as a soprano in college I have lost significant flexibility and range in my belt. As I exclusively study high soprano repertoire in voice lessons, and because life as a music education student is hectic and busy, I rarely have time to practice in my chest voice and have lost considerable skill. (Karin, written responses, p. 10)

Although Abbey, quoted above, expressed pride about being an alto, the participants mostly described connections between emotion and singing as negative, using expressions such as *fear, insecurity, pressure*, and *anxiety*. Emotional responses were largely triggered by preparation for a performance and the desire to please others, resulting in additional anxiety, self-consciousness, and frustration—and *guilt*. Our participants carried a great deal of guilt and insecurity with them. For example, one told us,

> Whenever I hear myself, like, on recordings, I always think it's not good enough. It's not full-enough sounding. It's not adult. It's not soprano-y enough sounding. It's not alto-y enough sounding. I'm very nitpicky; always have really high expectations for myself. I'm literally ready to run away from my jury. It's so scary. Like, "Oh what if I mess up? What if I don't sound good? What if the pitches are wrong?" (Ingrid, pp. 11–12)

Among our full recommendations and implications, Parker and I suggested the following for choral educators when helping female singers navigate voice change:

> We encourage teachers to select repertoire based on their singers' stage(s) of vocal development and re-voice as individual voices continue to evolve. Additional recommendations for choral settings include (a) maintaining an awareness of individual voices through frequent voice checks, (b) engaging in ongoing educational conversations with singers about vocal development, (c) varying choral singers' voice part assignment, and (d) carefully exercising the full vocal range in vocalises to encourage singers' emerging and individual vocal identities. (2018, p. 18)

Parker and I also endorsed the practice of encouraging females to develop their individual voices (as in opinions, attitudes, ideas, desires, so forth), both in and outside of choir. Key to this process was promoting (and applauding!) self-advocacy, especially within the choral setting:

> We recommend that music educators and voice teachers increase their awareness of women's self-identity development and adolescent women's tendencies to put the teacher and choir first and themselves second. Though teamwork is critical to identity development (see Parker, 2014), individuals must feel they are, in fact, important and contributing individuals to the team, whose ideas and perspectives are valued. Young women should feel empowered to self-advocate when necessary (Sweet, 2018). In studio and choral rehearsals, teachers should regularly solicit insight from vocalists about singing experiences. (Sweet & Parker, 2018, p. 18)

Since starting down this particular topical path of qualitative research, both solo and with my friend, it has been exciting to speak with many graduate students at different research venues who are also interested in the adolescent female voice. I look forward to their explorations come to fruition and entering professional conversations, advocating for females experiencing voice change and supporting the practices of choral music educators.

Honoring All Voices. It is common to have more females than males in choral programs, but that does not mean that females are well-served in choir or that choral programs are meeting females' musical, developmental, and personal needs. We cannot take our female students for granted, and it is time to invest in both female and male adolescent singers, especially those experiencing voice change. Here are some suggestions towards better meeting the needs of *all* our singers:

- First and foremost, honor and celebrate adolescent voice change for *all* singers, including females. Aim for the attitude that the glass is half full, not half empty. Is voice change always easy? Absolutely not, but celebrate successes and victories wherever you can! Such an approach establishes an important atmosphere in the choral classroom: Everyone is going through puberty, everyone is experiencing a voice change of some kind, everyone will work through elements of vocal adversity, and everyone will celebrate moments of vocal triumph. We are all in this together, regardless of sex or gender.
- Fight the stigma. As choral educators, we should overtly acknowledge female voice change and advocate more for female adolescent singers, both in our classrooms and in the larger profession. Embrace, promote, and celebrate it rather than fight, ignore, dread, and be frustrated by it.
- Discussions about adolescent voice change must be common occurrences in the choral classroom for two primary reasons:

    - Knowledge is power to adolescents. *Empower your singers!* When adolescents understand the physiological happenings with their voice, especially framed for both males and females, the entire experience seems much less scary and normal. As a result, students will more likely persevere through vocal challenges and continue singing.
    - Research has provided evidence that voice change can contribute to feelings of isolation for both males and females experiencing vocal challenges. In-class discussions that acknowledge and validate their experiences (and accompanying emotions) will assist all singers in feeling more supported throughout this developmental process.
- Inclusion of all students in discussions of voice change will only further substantiate the work that we do as choral music educators to students, parents, colleagues, and school administrators. By teaching

about the processes of the singing mechanism for all of our students, we strengthen our work as choral music educators and outwardly demonstrate our intentions to address the vocal needs of *all* of our adolescent choristers.

- Wield power *wisely*. As Voltaire said (although now associated with Uncle Ben from Spiderman), "With great power, comes great responsibility." Your students *trust you* and will do what you ask, regardless of what they believe might be best for themselves or want to try. Beware of an overabundance of ensemble-centric considerations and work to place the needs of all of your developing adolescent singers over the needs of the larger choir.
- If you are new to working with changing voices, remember that every age level requires you to consider *that* age level. During my years as a middle school teacher, some of my choir students began private voice lessons with a local voice teacher who was known for working with collegiate vocalists; occasionally this teacher would accept high school or middle school students. Despite sharing my concerns with the parents, my middle school students would launch head-first into all that I described earlier as "serious vocal work" with this renowned voice teacher—the first step of which was to be assigned to a specific voice part. The results were heartbreaking, for my adolescent singers quickly locked onto an identity as a specific voice part and began singing repertoire that required full, mature, sustained, powerful sounds not appropriate for their developing, wispy, fluctuating voices. Several struggled greatly in the following years, as their voices ultimately ended up sounding unnaturally mature and dark-vowel sounding for their age, which led to issues when blending with other singers in high school and beyond, as well as issues with vocal health. I am still at a loss as to why this voice teacher felt it was appropriate to teach those young people the same way he taught older students, but it proves that each voice must be approached according to the developmental needs of the individual. This leads me to the next point.
- Books of vocal exercises and warm-ups can be helpful in getting ideas to use with adolescent singers, but you *must* be critical of every exercise you read and make sure that it will serve *your* specific students well and support continued good vocal health. No one book of vocal exercises is going to suit all of your singers or all of your choirs; every voice, every choir is contextual, especially keeping in mind all that was discussed in chapter 1. However, now you are armed with understandings and holistic knowledge of the adolescent voice and singer from the many ideas within this book, and you can now truly scrutinize the many books of

vocal exercises available and find pedagogical techniques that best fit your unique students and choirs.

Meeting the needs of females with changing voices is similar to meeting the needs of their male counterparts. As music teachers and conductors, we must be overtly supportive. We must approach each student's voice change process individually and validate their physiological, mental, and emotional experiences. We must educate all of our singers about the voice change process, stressing the importance of healthy singing at all stages. Every one of our adolescent singers will pass through puberty at some point, and part of our job is to help our singers—both male and female—navigate vocal transitions and growth as smoothly as possible and as positively as possible.

RIOT ACTS

Several years ago, my former Illinois colleague, Louis Bergonzi, stopped me in the hallway and *excitedly* asked me, "Have you seen the documentary *Riot Acts* (2010)? It documents the stories of transgender professional musicians and there is a whole section on voice change. I think we could combine your interest on the adolescent changing voice with our shared interest of LGBTQ+ topics. Let's talk."

This conversation was the beginning of a multi-year project with Louis that focused on creating an instructional unit for middle school students around the documentary *Riot Acts*. The unit was designed to give adolescent music students insight and validation with regard to their own voice change and identity formation experiences from musical people who self-elect to go through voice change as part of their gender transition and self-realization process. In addition, through the unit we also wished to support LGBTQ+ students and allies in middle school music classes. Before I get too far ahead of myself, here is a description of *Riot Acts* from their website:

> *Riot Acts* is a "trans-fabulous" rockumentary representing the multi-faceted lives of transgender and gender variant musicians. A first-hand perspective of the intersections between gender performance and stage performance, *Riot Acts* suggests that identities and bodies are undeniably political, and the journey within a trans experience isn't always one of tragedy, but one of creativity and joy. (http://www.riotactsfilm.com/about.html)

This film received the Audience Choice Award at the 2011 TranScreen Film Festival in Amsterdam and won Best Documentary at the 2010 Philadelphia Independent Film Festival, the Audience Choice Award at the 2010 *Park City Film Music Festival*, and the Jury Award: Best Documentary at the 2009 Reeling Gay & Lesbian Film Festival.

Bergonzi and I developed a two-day unit and were proud to present it at the 2016 3rd Symposium on LGBT Studies and Music Education, the 2016 32nd World Conference of the International Society for Music Education in Glasgow, Scotland, and the 2016 Illinois Music Education Association All-State Conference (Sweet & Bergonzi, 2016a; Sweet & Bergonzi, 2016b; Sweet, Martin, & Bergonzi, 2016). The support we received for our work was incredibly encouraging; the tricky part, however, was finding a school or district that would allow us to teach the unit to their middle school students. After countless (and I do mean *countless*) roadblocks, last-minute rejections, meetings with school officials, Institutional Review Board revisions, and appeals to music educators, we were granted permission to present our instructional unit to seventh and eighth graders at a private middle school in Chicago; we were also granted permission to collect research data about the experience. I'll cut right to the chase: Although we were fully supported by the administration, faculty, and staff of the middle school, and supported by a few parents in this very progressive setting, hardly any students agreed to participate, and those who did elected not to complete the materials we created for data collection. Here is what I wrote to the wonderful principal and music teacher on our behalf after analyzing data:

> We've been through all of the collected data and, unfortunately, do not have enough data to move forward towards a publication or presentation of the project. The participant pool was quite small and from that pool only one student provided responses/information on only one of the questionnaires. With only three short student interview transcripts and one questionnaire, we concede at this time. (Sweet & Bergonzi, email to the principal and teacher, 2017)

It was an absolutely heartbreaking way to end the study that we had worked years to make happen. However, every experience is a learning experience.

I have grown incredibly fond of *Riot Acts* and now share the section on voice change with my choral methods students every year. Based on Internet searches, I don't know that many of the bands featured in the documentary are still together, but the documentary is like a wonderfully preserved time capsule of transgender perspective. It is fascinating to hear about voice change from adults with adult vocabularies and adult understandings of the world. Adolescents tend to not be so great at verbalizing how they feel about what is going on, but these musicians are very articulate when describing their voice change experiences, their fears, their successes, and the role that their voice plays in who they are as people and musicians. I think that in the right context, sharing (edited) clips from this documentary with adolescents would enable them to better realize and verbalize their own voice change experiences, validate their frustrations and challenges, and empower them through this process.

In this day and age, choral teachers are working with students who openly identify as transgender or gender expansive more and more, and such developments are leading choral educators to consider different ways to best work with their singers. Some students may be preparing for or already involved in hormone therapy, which has implications in the choral classroom; some students may not be planning to start hormone therapy but strongly identify with a voice part that is quite different from their physiological voice; or some students may identify with a different gender but want to continue singing the voice part that most aligns with their physiological voice. Over the past several years, whenever I have presented a conference session or workshop on the changing voice to middle or high school choral teachers, inevitably someone asks me a question about a specific singer in their choir who identifies as transgender. My response always includes encouragement to ensure that the student is constantly maintaining good vocal health, but each scenario is unique and I give my insight on a case-by-case basis. I do often include the following story, however: I was fortunate to see a music conference session a few years ago that featured a panel of high school students comprised of two lesbians, a gay male, and two transgender students. The students spoke of their experiences as LGBTQ+ students in music and allowed the teacher attendees to ask many, many questions. The question-and-answer period pretty much went like this:

TEACHER #1: I have a student who openly identifies [rest of brief story]. What should I do?

STUDENT PANEL: Have you spoken to the student to find out what they need or would like?

TEACHER #1: No, I haven't.

STUDENT PANEL: You should talk with your student.

TEACHER #2: I have a student who openly identifies [rest of brief story]. What should I do?

STUDENT PANEL: Have you spoken to the student to find out what they need or would like?

TEACHER #2: No, I haven't.

STUDENT PANEL: You should talk with your student.

TEACHER #3: I have a student who openly identifies [rest of brief story]. What should I do?

STUDENT PANEL: Have you spoken to the student to find out what they need or would like?

TEACHER #3: No, I haven't.

STUDENT PANEL: You should talk with your student.

Finally, the panel members blatantly said to the audience, "If your student is open about their identity and you want to know what they need, then *talk with your student*." A core intention of this book is to encourage choral educators to empower adolescents to speak up and ask questions about their vocal challenges and to have a voice throughout that process. That should not be any different when working with students who identify as transgender. All adolescents have a voice, and our job as music educators is to help them realize and actualize it, literally and figuratively.

This conversation also directly connects with the topic of voice classification systems. Because their voice is such an integral part of their identity, transgender students often do not want to be assigned a voice classification that does not align with their personal identity. While there is not space in this book to fully unpack the anatomy, physiology, and pedagogy of transgender voices, at the end of this chapter I provide a few suggestions for working with adolescent voices beyond classification systems; these suggestions also support students who identify as transgender. It is highly likely that each of us will work with a student who identifies as transgender several times during our music teaching career. Some students will be very open about it during our time together, but some will not reveal this facet of themselves for many more years. The bottom line is, working with all students graciously and encouragingly is hugely important, as is modeling nurturance, support, and advocacy for each of your students.

What follows is a transcript of the section of *Riot Acts* (2010) that addressed transgender voice change. This documentary is especially compelling when you hear the musicians speak their own words and perform their own music throughout, so I strongly encourage you to watch the actual documentary sometime (available via Amazon Video).

As you read, I charge you with a prompt from the study that Louis and I developed; this prompt is similar to what we asked of our middle school research participants:

Think about the way that these transgender musicians describe their voice change and compare or contrast with your own voice change experiences (or experiences working with changing voice adolescents). How have your experiences with voice change been similar or different to those of the transgender musicians in *Riot Acts*?

While contemplating these musicians' comments, notice what comes up for you with regard to how you currently interact with all of your adolescent singers, knowing that some of them may identify as transgender at some point in their lives.

As you read, bear in mind that (1) the word *testosterone* is often referenced as *T* in the transcript and (2) there is some salty language; Louis and I created edited clips of this movie for our research with the middle school students with permission from the documentary's director.

<begin transcript>

There is hardly a moment throughout this section where music is not heard or where the featured artist is not shown singing a song in a variety of performance contexts. What follows is the conversation as presented in this section of the documentary *Riot Acts*.

Those featured first in this section on voice change are female to male (FTM) transgender musicians. They now identify as male.

RYDER RICHARDSON

When I hear recordings of my voice, I'm a little disturbed. I'm like, "Ah! I sound so feminine!" And that's not how I *think* I sound. And I think a lot of the time I do sing lower. And I think I limit my range because I'm not comfortable singing in a higher voice and sometimes I think that's kind of limiting.

Singer from the band *THE CLIKS*

You know, it's weird. I don't think it was really a very conscious thing that I did think about my voice. From the albums that I had before where

I was solo, I was identifying as female and when I listen to my voice *now*, I kind of feel like my voice is deepened and these guys (*gestures towards two other bandmates sitting there as well*) would agree with me because I feel like I'm losing my high end and I complain about it all the time. And I'm *not* on testosterone and I'm not planning on doing that any time soon because I know that it *will* affect my voice, or *apparently* it will. And I don't really want to risk that.

ADHAMH ROLAND

(a very worried look on his face) If I'm on T, *what the hell is my voice going to sound like?! Music is such a big part of my life! Like, what if I can't sing anymore?!* Or like, what is it going to be like in the first couple . . . maybe, even *years* of taking T if that ever happens? And people come to shows and what is my public identity going to be like?

GEO WYETH, A.K.A *NOVICE THEORY*

In terms of building my career as an artist, you really want somebody to hear your voice and say, "That's *that person!* That's Geo!" That's not mysterious, who's singing right now. But if your voice is changing, it's challenging. (*a long clip of him singing to an audience while accompanying himself on an accordion*)

ANDERSON TOONE

One of the things that kept me from taking T for all the years--I started transitioning at [age] 45. . . I'm gonna be [age] 49 on Tuesday--and I would have probably started 10-15 years earlier, but I heard a lot of myths and believed them that my voice would be destroyed.

JOE STEPHENS from the band *COYOTE GRACE*

My voice was my first instrument, guitar sort of came second. My voice was the main thing. I was a soprano. I asked doctors and other trans guys, "Like, is it going to be okay? Am I still going to be able to sing?" And everyone was like (*shrugs his shoulders upwards*), "Eh? We don't know." Because there's just not a lot study on it and not enough people have gone through it.

ELIJAH OBERMAN from the band *THE SHONDES*

Being worried about whether I was going to be able to sing really affected *how* I transitioned and doing things very gradually and slowly that actually allows your vocal cords to adjust at a more gradual pace instead of being *shocked* into a certain place.

JOE STEPHENS from the band *COYOTE GRACE*

I couldn't not go on T. So that was the end of that.

The main singer from the band *TOUGH TOUGH SKIN*

I had this very well-trained sort of second soprano/alto-type voice and then starting T was kind of like walking in the woods. You don't know *what's* going to happen. It was like, "Okay! It's cracking! It's cracking on stage! It sounds great!" But I guess I just kind of worked with it. "Okay! We're gonna yodel! Today we're gonna yodel."

Those featured in this next section on voice change are male to female (MTF) transgender musicians. They now identify as female.

RYKA AOKI

I've known so many guys who take the testosterone and their voice drops. And many of them are musicians and singers. And how does one develop a new voice because that voice is dropping, I'm sorry, that voice is dropping. For trans women, we don't get the . . . updraft. (*long pause*) But how can *we* sing?

SHAWNA LOVE from the band *LIPSTICK CONSPIRACY*

You know, we're all singing and stuff and I'm going through my head, "Oh my God, we sound like a bunch of lumberjacks!" But you know, but that's not something that we're ever gonna change or even begin to worry about. We sound like we sound. And I'm not about to even *go there*. It just is what it is. And so I thought, "Okay." And I was still uncomfortable with it. I didn't like it. I didn't like the way we sounded. I didn't like our harmony--it sounded like *male* harmony. Especially when I'd seen some other trans people who had done some sort of vocal coaching or lessons or whatever. And they sound *completely feminine*. I was like, "Oh! I want to sound like that!" But that wasn't the case for us. That was something that I had to come to terms with.

JESSICA XAVIER

I wanted to sing in an alto range. I wanted to get up there and try and reach that. I was going through speech therapy at the same time that I was taking lessons with a voice coach. And she was getting me to work on this, what she called, an alto-falsetto blend. I was totally in denial about how testosterone had destroyed my Vienna Choirboy perfect voice.

The rest of this section of the documentary features all the musicians, regardless of identification as a transgender woman or man.

The three members of the band *SYSTYR ACT*

[The members of Systyr Act describe their band as a "nun cover band" and perform rock songs dressed as Catholic nuns.]

BAND MEMBER #1: You're *a nun* singing. You're not Greg, Tam, Travis. You're *Sister*.

BAND MEMBER #2: I'm *glorifying God with my voice.* It doesn't matter how I sound dressed as a nun singing rock covers.

BAND MEMBER #1: *Amen.*

MAILE THIESEN and KELLY MOE of the band
BASIC FIX

MAILE (speaking about her transgender male bandmate, Kelly): People listen to the recording and a lot of times people don't get it that Kelly's the singer, even though his face is on there and it says it's produced *all* by him and he made everything . . . but people are like, "Who's that girl that's singing on your album?" Like, *all the time* people ask that. And he's like, "It's me," and they're like, "What?!" And they'll say, "Do you change your voice to sound like that?"

KELLY: They will ask me, "Do you tweak it?" (*making a gesture indicating turning a knob to make an electronic adjustment of his voice*) And I don't.

KRISTEN ANCHOR and RAHNE ALEXANDER of the band
THE DEGENERETTES

KRISTEN (to Rahne, who has a higher-sounding voice): You've said before to me that you've kind of lucked out in that you didn't have to make a decision to modulate your voice like some other trans women that you know have said they *had* to do in order to feel comfortable. Luck of the draw there, right?

RAHNE: Yeah, definitely. I feel it is the luck of the draw! Any *real work* that I've done on my voice in terms of singing, I think it's the same as anybody else who's singing. It's just really learning to use it in the context of the songs that are being presented and trying to make my voice match that.

RYKA AOKI

So much of it is intonation and play rather than actual pitch. There are some female singers who have much deeper voices than either of us do. I think sometimes we get too hung up on pitch as opposed to intonation and cadence and all that sort of goodness.

ELIJAH OBERMAN from the band *THE SHONDES*

Being able to sing is part of my identity. And I think that more than anything scared me to death about transitioning.

GEO WYETH, A.K.A *NOVICE THEORY*

All I know is I decided at a certain point after being very afraid for a while going, "I'm not going to be able to sing! I'm not going to be able to sing!" I thought, you know what? I'm just gonna do it and *I'm gonna sing.*

JOE STEPHENS from the band *COYOTE GRACE*

It was sort of day-job-in-Seattle time of my life--it wasn't thrilling--but I just stayed home and sang and I sang through it and it squeaked and my range *shrunk*! And then it got down on the bottom and it slowly starting to go up. So I was dealing with a *fifth* of a range, which was *significantly* smaller than what it was before! (*laughing*) And all of my songs changed *keys*--I had a *huge* body of work--and all my songs changed keys! It finally went around to where I dropped almost an octave, so they are almost back in the same key where they were.

It's muscle memory, so your larynx and all the muscles in your throat, you know, they think, "I know how to hit that note! We do *this* . . ." And then it's not that note anymore! So basically, it's like somebody restrung my guitar and I just have to figure out where the new notes are.

ELIJAH OBERMAN from the band *THE SHONDES*
When you can't hear yourself but you know that you're singing on key because you know how a note feels in your throat and it's *not* anymore . . .

JOE STEPHENS from the band *COYOTE GRACE*
And it's a different emotive quality to the voice which is interesting to get used to. I feel like I'm very blessed to have been born in this time when transition and hormones are available. I'm very happy with my body now; I'm very happy with my voice. And that's great. The *loss* (*pause*) is those *soaring* treble notes that I could just sort of *wail* at any moment's notice. It was a *different feeling* that was being conveyed and I could just . . . every once in a while I still think I can sing them and I (*mouths a word, but no sound comes out*), but (*laughing*) it's not there!

Joe, singing with his guitar on stage while his bandmate, Ingrid Elizabeth, plays the upright bass:

Who am I to change my life?
Who am I to fuck with form?
Who am I to weather the storm?
But I go slow.
I said goodbye to everyone I know.
And one morning I awoke,
And I was this guy named Joe.

INGRID ELIZABETH from the band COYOTE GRACE
Yeah, I sang with him when he was a soprano and, yes, he had those beautiful soaring high notes but this is such a truer expression of who he is and where he comes from and his experience and just his truest self. And that, in itself, is beautiful.

ANDERSON TOONE
The richness of having it where I want it and also some of the other gender congruencies of becoming

more masculine is SO satisfying. . . . [next sentence omitted] This congruency that I now have is worth having to change the key or even having to say goodbye to certain tunes or my role in them or whatever, man.

SARAFINA MARASCHINO of the band LIPSTICK CONSPIRACY

It was interesting to suddenly have to recognize, "I'm a girl now. I'm in a girl band. I'm singing as a girl." I'm not trying to fool anybody and the idea of somebody saying, "Well you don't really sound like a girl, though . . ." And it's like (looking bewildered), "Well, what is . . . hmmm . . . SO?" We know what we are and we know what we're not so it's like, "Yeah, I agree." This is how I sing. And this is how I speak. I've got a low voice. And for the longest time it was like, yeah, I was the baritone in the band so I still am kinda, I guess. But whatever. Yeah, so what?

GEO WYETH, A.K.A NOVICE THEORY

Going from singing these songs from before I was on hormones and now singing them now--and I still do, I play all the time--but it's . . . it's hard. And then I hear my CD that I sell, which is all tracks of me before I started hormones. And people have said to me, "I can't believe that's you!" It's wild. People come see my shows and they're like, "You used to sound so incredibly different." And it's true, I do. It's sort of painful for me to acknowledge that because it scares me and makes me think, well, maybe people won't want to buy my music now or people liked my voice before better or they like it more now. . . or . . .

<end transcript>

If we consider what the musicians featured in *Riot Acts* said about their voices, three major themes emerged: *vocal challenges, fear of the unknown*, and *we all have our own voice*. Vocal challenges included cracking or the inability to sing certain pitches or acceptance that today was yodeling day. I appreciated Joe's comment comparing his voice change to someone having restrung his guitar, and that he had to just figure out where the new notes were—what a great, accessible analogy. To complicate matters for these singers, not only did vocal challenges affect technical manipulations of the voice, but they impacted musicians' abilities to express emotive qualities, which is a powerful consideration. Not only was the *how I express myself* affected, the *what I can express* was affected too.

My heart went out to the musicians whenever they discussed fear of the unknown with their voices: how will this process unfold? Will I be able to sing in the end? Is everything going to be okay? I am always struck by Geo's wondering if people will like his voice more before voice change or after voice change. The unknown is scary enough when just considering acquiring an entirely new voice; it is a new level of intensity when adding worry about other people's opinions to the mix.

Whenever I watch *Riot Acts* I am very impressed with the musicians' attitudes about their voices, both with regard to their voice change and just in general. The messages that "we all have our own voice" and "this is *my voice*" come through loud and clear, regardless of characteristics of their voices or whether or not they experienced a voice change. Ultimately, all of these singers and musicians sought to actualize their "truest self" and, regardless of what their voice sounds like, they are rock-solid regarding who they are as people and as expressive musicians. A lot of what was said absolutely aligns with how adolescents with changing voices have described their singing experiences and what we hope for them. While I understand that each teaching situation has its own unique challenges, I encourage you to ponder ways to bring these transgender musicians' voices into your conversations with students about their adolescent voice change. Honor and validation come in many shapes and forms and, for many reasons, perspective from the musicians in *Riot Acts* may be exactly what some of your adolescent students need to hear in order for them to feel empowered to sing.

DIGEST

I stated very clearly at the beginning of this book that its purpose was not to provide warm-ups or lists of repertoire to use with singers with changing voices. My reasoning is that each voice and each choir is unique, and my recommendations may not be the best fit for the context of your choral program. It is up to individual choral educators to determine how best to meet the needs of their own choirs and singers. That said, with all discussed in this chapter in mind, I would like to suggest a few ideas for working with changing voices beyond classification systems, especially with regard to approaching repertoire. There are certain characteristics of pieces of music that work really well with changing voices as you help students hone their skills, and once you learn to identify such details, the options for choral repertoire increase exponentially.

- Songs with independent parts work well with adolescent changing voices. When the parts are different enough from each other, students are less likely to get "sucked into" the other vocal parts (a common problem for changing voices; see chapters 1 and 2 again for some reasons why).
- Similarly, parallels can be tricky to hold. When I was a new teacher, I thought that holding a third throughout a song would be easy for my junior high singers; it was just a third, after all! I soon realized that staying on one's own part can be extremely tricky for certain changing voices. This doesn't mean that students should not be taught to hold parts against one another, but songs with more independent parts rather than lots of parallel movement will help them to be more successful right away.
- As male voices begin to drop and are trapped between treble clef and bass clef, it is okay for them to flip octaves up or down if they are unable to access an entire vocal line as written. I have found that the flip typically takes place around F or G both below and above middle C. If you teach your students how to do this themselves, they can automatically mark octave flips in their music and you can just check in with them to see what they are planning to do in their part rather than keeping track of everyone yourself. When adolescent singers understand their voice and the tools available to help them be successful musicians in the moment, they can self-advocate in many ways that help you fulfill your mission as a music educator: to foster musical independence. As male voices continue to lower in pitch, flipping the octave will become moot and they will eventually be able to sing most notes in their lower developing vocal range.
- Moving the overall key of a piece up or down a half step can solve a great many tuning issues. Case in point: Last summer, my Illinois Summer Youth Music Junior Chorus was singing a piece written in the key of F Major. We had tuning issue after tuning issue after tuning issue, no matter what I did to help students sing in tune. Because I was graced with an accompanist who could transpose music on the spot, I had the students try the piece in F# major and it was *gloriously* in tune! Not one single issue remained. The choir sang the song in tune forevermore in

F# and we never returned to F. While I have been unable to find research to support this practice, it may work because of how keys fit and feel differently in students' registers; perhaps it is simply a novelty effect, in that singing feels and sounds somewhat different, and students hone in on what they are doing more effectively as they perk up; or perhaps it has something to do with brain re-wiring and the ability to interpret some sounds more effectively than others. Regardless of why or how this works, it is a good strategy with changing voices.

- An SSA arrangement might work infinitely better with a specific group of changing voices than the SAB arrangement of the same piece. Examine both when researching new music.
- Unison pieces can be amazing with middle-level singers of like voices, such as all treble or all bass. They can be used to teach singers about phrasing, breath control, expression, and tuning. That said, unison music can be extremely challenging for changing voices as the vocal lines cannot be sung without flipping octaves. No one wants to flip octaves throughout an entire piece of music; it's boring and frustrating. Rather, save unison pieces for adolescent voices that are either completely together in one vocal range or completely aligned in different octaves; find a different piece with multiple parts to honor the voices at various stages of change.
- Instead of forcing a round peg into a square hole, you may need to rearrange the square. Do not be afraid to rearrange a small section of a piece of music to assist your singers. Keep them singing, even if that means creating a little alternate version of a vocal line to sing. *Do not tell them to stop singing if they cannot hit the notes.* Adolescents could mistakenly interpret "do not sing here" as "I can't sing, the teacher said so." Proceed with caution and care.
- Keep all adolescents singing throughout their entire range, and move singers between melodic and harmonic vocal parts often—especially treble voices. Choral professor Judy Bowers wrote about this in "Building Early Choral Experiences: Part Two—The Middle School Choral Program" when discussing soprano and alto voice parts (in your choir it could include unchanged male voices as well as female voices): Each part can rotate between soprano and alto throughout the year. Those who resist alto because they can hear the melody and sing it quickly will be unhappy when it is their turn to provide the harmony, and those who prefer alto because the soprano range is uncomfortable (read: no head tone) will be unhappy when they must sing the high notes; but, with time, all the girls will gain skill in using the entire range (generally one and a half octaves, perhaps D to high A), plus all will be learning

to maintain melody and harmony, even while they are learning to read music and sing with beautiful tone. (2008, p. 364)

I appreciate Bowers's commentary, as I firmly believe that our work as choral music educators involves fostering development of a student's entire instrument. Supporting adolescents through voice change might mean that some of them sing parts that they do not want to try, resulting in their being annoyed or frustrated with us, their teachers. The way I see it, if we are damned if we do (broaden their experiences and develop their skills) and damned if we don't (let them sing what is most comfortable and not step outside the physiologically dictated comfort zone), I would rather have a student frustrated with me for embracing my role as a music educator, which results in their gaining new skills and learning from new musical experiences. How *you* proceed in your classroom is entirely up to you.

- Special touches in a piece of music matter, as they keep it interesting. Insist on that dynamic contrast or rhythmic vitality! The choir may not always sing a song perfectly in tune, but it can control details that keep the music exciting, interesting, and captivating. They just have to understand the importance of such details and be held accountable for them.
- Personal investment in a song *matters greatly*, no matter the song, no matter the message, no matter the composer, era, style, or genre. If adolescent singers do not feel a connection to a piece of music, they will likely disengage. Our work includes providing discussion and connections between the music and the adolescent singers, encouraging personal threads of commonality with or in opposition to a piece of music, helping students develop emotional responses to choral music (whatever they may be) and allowing time and a welcome space to unpack and interpret those responses.

Reimagining the music is an important part of working with adolescent singers. In what ways can you navigate musical pieces to help your specific changing voice singers gain skill and confidence to continue singing? Do not feel limited by the predetermined voicings indicated on a piece of music when working with changing voices. If a student's voice works best with the notes of the soprano line but they have a bass voice, try the student on the soprano line down an octave. If you have an overabundance of treble voices and a dearth of bass voices, have half of the treble singers sing the bass line up an octave. Perhaps have groups of treble and bass voices on each part, some of whom will sing in unison in places in the song and sing in octaves in other places. It is imperative to consider singers' individual voices and help them successfully gain control of their instrument through vocal lines that will challenge them but also help them feel accomplished. I also encourage the act of identifying groups in the choir by the part they are singing on a piece of music as opposed to by personal identification with a specific voice part. The instruction "On this song you are singing alto" is much different from telling students "You are an alto."

At the University of Illinois, we have 27 different one-week camps during the summer as part of our Illinois Summer Youth Music program. Each summer I conduct the Junior Chorus, which involves students from sixth to eighth grade, and quite often the singers are somewhere in the midst of voice change. The camp is organized so that the students declare a voice part when they enter Junior Chorus for the week: soprano, alto, tenor, or bass. I typically choose around five pieces for the choir to learn during the week (prior to knowing the composition of the choir), which include:

- A trio of three-part or four-part songs to learn via the voicings by which students categorized themselves at the start of the week.
- One song for which I reimagine the voices so that there are mixed groups on all of the vocal lines. This fosters a nice community because students are singing next to new people. It also helps them work on listening and tuning skills.
- One song for which I have all of the students sing all of the parts and then choose the line they want to sing. The only rule is that, when all is said and done, the parts have to be balanced volume-wise. It always works out *beautifully*. Reasons behind students' decisions about which part to sing cover the gamut, but more than anything the students love the autonomy associated with choosing what they get to sing. They love having a literal voice over their figurative voice, and it is nice to provide them a little power over their voices during our week together.

Benefits of reimagining the music for singers with changing voices are many. Such teaching practices help students avoid locking onto the identity of one specific voice part prior to the conclusion of physiological growth of their instrument. It breaks down stigmas associated with specific voice parts in choir, such as the idea that only girls follow the treble line or only boys follow the bass line; this can be enormously helpful for that one male soprano or alto. If we diminish stigmas about voice parts, students may be less likely to limit their own voices by following what specific voice parts stereotypically can and cannot do (e.g, sopranos cannot sing low or altos cannot sing high). When you reconceptualize music based on your students, those in your choir who identify as gender expansive or as transgender can sing vocal lines that better align with their personal identity. As students wait for their voices to settle, they can continually develop their music reading and listening skills by following alternate vocal lines and listening for different harmonies or octaves around them. By exploring different singer combinations or vocal lines, you also give students opportunities to sing more closely with different people in their choir rather than only singing with those who share a voice part. I am sure that you are able to think of many more benefits beyond these few.

In closing, changing voices are not always the most accurate, not always the prettiest-sounding, not always the most versatile, but I find them to be some of the most sincere and endearing sounds on the planet. Working with adolescents and changing voices is not about perfection but about kindness, perseverance, understanding, patience, forward motion, celebration of all the successes, and a sense of humor. There will always be room for improvement and further growth, both musically and personally, but helping singers with changing voices to be successful in any ways they can be is one of the *best* parts of our job as choral music teachers.

ADDITIONAL RESOURCES

This section is intended to identify additional items that may further enhance or enrich your exploration of topics discussed in this book. Citations for publications discussed in each chapter can be found in the References section.

CHAPTER 1

For more insight into adolescence, development, and brain-related matters:

- Barrett, K. C., Ashley, R., Strait, D. L., & Kraus, N. (2013). Art and science: How musical training shapes the brain. *Frontiers in Psychology, 4*, article 713.
- Hammond, Z. (2015). *Culturally responsive teaching and the brain: Promoting authentic engagement and rigor among culturally and linguistically diverse students.* Thousand Oaks, CA: Sage.
- McNeely, C., & Blanchard, J. (2009). *The teen years explained: A guide to healthy adolescent development.* Baltimore: Center for Adolescent Health at the Johns Hopkins Bloomberg School of Public Health.
- Project AWARE: "All Project AWARE programs support teens telling real life stories in a powerful way. Young people create high quality movies that address social issues and make a difference." www.projectaware.net
- Skoe, E., & Kraus, N. (2013). Musical training heightens auditory brainstem function during sensitive periods in development. *Frontiers in Psychology, 4*, article 622.
- Tierney, A., Krizman, J., Skoe, E., Johnston, K., & Kraus, N. (2013). High school music classes enhance the neural processing of speech. *Frontiers in Psychology, 4*, article 855.
- Writings about adolescence by Kathleen Stassen Berger, John W. Santrock, and Laurence Steinberg (www.laurencesteinberg.com)

Resources regarding adolescent mental health:

- The Anxiety and Depression Society of America (https://adaa.org/living-with-anxiety/children)
- National Alliance on Mental Illness: Teens and Young Adults (https://www.nami.org/Find-Support/Teens-and-Young-Adults)
- National Institute of Mental Health: Teen Depression (https://www.nimh.nih.gov/health/publications/teen-depression/index.shtml)
- National Institute of Mental Health: Anxiety Disorders (https://www.nimh.nih.gov/health/topics/anxiety-disorders/index.shtml)
- Substance Abuse and Mental Health Services Administration: Help and Treatment (https://www.samhsa.gov/find-help)

CHAPTER 2

Additional resources on vocal anatomy and physiology:

- Abitol, J. (2019). *The female voice*. San Diego: Plural Publishing.
- Bastian Voice Institute: http://www.bastianvoice.com/2010/07/capillary-ectasia-ce/.
- Callaghan, J. (2000). *Singing and voice science*. San Diego: Singular Publishing Group.
- Gunjawate, D. R., Aithal, V. U., Ravi, R., & Venkatesh, B. T. (2017). The effect of menstrual cycle on singing voice: A systematic review. *Journal of Voice, 31*(2), 188–194.
- Hari Kumar, K. V. S., Garg, A., Ajai Chandra, N. S., Singh, S. P., & Datta, R. (2016). Voice and endocrinology. *Indian Journal of Endocrinology and Metabolism, 20*, 590–594.
- Heman-Ackah, Y. D., Sataloff, R. T., & Hawkshaw, M. J. (2013). *The voice: A medical guide for achieving and maintaining a healthy voice*. Narberth, PA: Science & Medicine.
- Jahn, A., & Blitzer, A. (1996). A short history of laryngoscopy. *Logopedics, Phoniatrics, Vocology, 21*, 181–185.
- Ravens, S. (2014). *The supernatural voice: A history of high male singing*. Woodbridge, Suffolk, UK: Boydell Press.
- Roers, F., Mürbe, D., & Sundberg, J. (2009). Voice classification and vocal tract of singers: A study of x-ray images and morphology. *Journal of the Acoustical Society of America, 125*(1), 503–512.

- Scherer, R. C. (2014). Laryngeal function during phonation. In J. S. Rubin, R. T. Sataloff, & G. S. Korovin (Eds.), *Diagnosis and treatment of voice disorders* (4th ed., pp. 117–144). San Diego: Plural Publishing.
- Sundberg, J. (1987). *The Science of the Singing Voice.* DeKalb: Northern Illinois University Press.
- Wicklund, K. (2010). *Singing voice rehabilitation: A guide for the voice teacher and speech language pathologist.* Clifton Park, NY: Delmar.

CHAPTER 3

Resources for promoting empathy, kindness, and community in choral classrooms:

- Editors of Conari Press. (2013). *Random acts of kindness: Then and now.* Berkeley, CA: Conari Press.
- Emdin, C. (2017). *For white folks who teach in the hood . . . and the rest of y'all too: Pedagogy and urban education (race, education, and democracy).* Boston: Beacon Press.
- Howe, D. (2013). *Empathy: What it is and why it matters.* New York: Palgrave Macmillan.
- Ladson-Billings, G. (2009). *The Dreamkeepers: Successful teachers of African American children* (2nd ed.). San Francisco, CA: Jossey-Bass.
- Lind, V. R., & McKoy, C. L. (2016). *Culturally responsive teaching in music education: From understanding to application.* New York: Routledge.
- Maddi, S. R. (2013). *Hardiness: Turning stressful circumstances into resilient growth.* New York: Springer.
- Malin, H., Teilly, T. S., Quinn, B., & Moran, S. (2013). Adolescent purpose development: Exploring empathy, discovering roles, shifting priorities, and creating pathways. *Journal of Research on Adolescence, 24*(1), 186–199.
- Sensoy, Ö., & DiAngelo, R. (2017). *Is everyone really equal?: An introduction to key concepts in social justice education* (2nd ed.). New York: Teaches College Press.
- Sweet, B. (2010). A case study: Middle school boys' perceptions of singing and participation in choir. *Update: Applications of Research in Music Education, 28*(2), 5–12.
- Talbot, B. C. (Ed.). (2018). *Marginalized voices in music education.* New York: Routledge.

- Toulis, J. (2011). Teaching children empathy. In A. N. Johnson & M. W. Neagley (Eds.), *Educating from the heart: Theoretical and practical approaches to transforming education* (pp. 127–136). Lanham, MD: Rowman & Littlefield Education.
- Tyink, S. (2008, Jan). Teaching empathy to young adolescents: Suggestions for building empathy in the middle grades (Developmental Designs article). Retrieved from http://www.originsonline.org/newsletters/winter-2008-dd/teaching-empathy-young-adolescents

Further information about ideas within *Grit*, as well as initial reviews of the book:

- Angela Duckworth's website: https://angeladuckworth.com/
- Angela Duckworth's TED Talk on ideas from *Grit*: https://www.ted.com/talks/angela_lee_duckworth_grit_the_power_of_passion_and_perseverance
- *New York Times* review of *Grit* by Judith Shulevitz: https://www.nytimes.com/2016/05/08/books/review/grit-by-angela-duckworth.html
- *Forbes* article, "5 characteristics of grit: How many do you have?" by Margaret M. Perlis https://www.forbes.com/sites/margaretperlis/2013/10/29/5-characteristics-of-grit-what-it-is-why-you-need-it-and-do-you-have-it/#5b8f8cdf4f7b
- *National Geographic* article, "Grit trumps talent and IQ: A story every parent (and educator) should read," by Marguerite Del Giudice https://news.nationalgeographic.com/news/2014/10/141015-angela-duckworth-success-grit-psychology-self-control-science-nginnovators/
- National Public Radio interview with Angela Duckworth, "Forget Talent, Success Comes From 'Grit,'" by Rachel Martin https://www.npr.org/2016/05/01/476346709/forget-talent-success-comes-from-grit

Critical reviews of *Grit*:

- Credé, M. (2018). What shall we do about grit? A critical review of what we know and what we don't know. *Educational Researcher, 47*(9), 606–611.
- National Public Radio feature, "MacArthur 'Genius' Angela Duckworth responds to a new critique of *Grit*," by Anya Kamenetz https://www.npr.org/sections/ed/2016/05/25/479172868/angela-duckworth-responds-to-a-new-critique-of-grit

- *New Yorker* article, "The limits of 'Grit,'" by David Denby https://www.newyorker.com/culture/culture-desk/the-limits-of-grit
- *Washington Post* article, "The problem with teaching 'grit' to poor kids? They already have it. Here's what they really need," by Valerie Strauss https://www.washingtonpost.com/news/answer-sheet/wp/2016/05/10/the-problem-with-teaching-grit-to-poor-kids-they-already-have-it-heres-what-they-really-need/?utm_term=.97a3a92a7615
- *Wall Street Journal* opinion article, "Is there anything grit can't do?" by Kay S. Hymowitz https://www.wsj.com/articles/is-there-anything-grit-cant-do-1498254238

CHAPTER 4

Additional media portrayals of voice change:

- *Bye Bye Birdie*
  In the 1963 movie version of the American musical *Bye Bye Birdie*, the song "The Telephone Hour" features Harvey Johnson (played by Peter Menefee) as the nerdy teenager clearly experiencing a voice change. Harvey Johnson experiences unfortunate voice cracks at about 1:00, again at around 2:00, and again at 2:22 minutes.
- *Supernatural*
  In *Supernatural*, two brothers fight evil supernatural beings of many kinds, including monsters, demons, and gods that roam the earth. In the episode "Teen Dean" (season 10, episode 12) Dean goes back to his adolescent self and experiences puberty all over again, but with an adult mind during the process.
- *Leave It to Beaver*
  During season 5 of *Leave It to Beaver*, the voice of Jerry Mathers, the actor who played Beaver Cleaver, varied quite a lot. It is pretty evident that the actor was experiencing voice change during this particular season, although it was not a part of the storyline for Beaver (as it was for Adam in *The Goldbergs*, as discussed in chapter 4).
- *The Simpsons*
  Season 4, episode 11 of *The Simpsons* (1992), titled "Homer's Triple Bypass," gives a nice nod to Homer's adolescent voice change. In this part of the episode, young Homer Simpson is beautifully singing "O Holy Night" in a lilting high soprano voice in front of a huge church crowd, as his father watches from a pew in the congregation:

HOMER'S FATHER

What a voice! Young Homer's going to make me a millionaire!

YOUNG HOMER

Oh, night . . . di- *(crack, squeak, low squawk and a very low out-of-tune voice takes over)* VINE. Hey! My voice just changed!

HOMER'S FATHER

Dang nab it!

The Simpsons also features a reoccurring character known simply as "Squeaky-Voiced Teen," whose voice breaks and cracks from high to low as his talks. A good example is in "Lisa vs. Malibu Stacy" (season 5, episode 14), where Squeaky-Voiced Teen is working as a fast-food manager and his voice pitches and cracks back and forth from high to low as he instructs his employees:

SQUEAKY-VOICED TEEN

(high and squeaky) We need some more secret *(voice cracks low)* sauce! *(voice cracks between high and low)* Put this mayonnaise in the sun!

- *Family Guy*
  Another adult animated show, *Family Guy*, also briefly featured main character Peter's voice change in "Believe It or Not, Joe's Walking on Air" (season 5, episode 3). In this very fast cut-away scene, Peter is talking to two friends in an extremely high, unchanged voice—until he reaches the last syllable of the sentence, when his voice suddenly drops into bass territory and he walks away with a changed voice:

PETER

(high, unchanged voice) Hey, you guys feeling like playing some base- *(voice suddenly drops dramatically low)* BALL?

- *Diary of a Wimpy Kid* (2010)
  Greg Heffley, age 12, tells the story of his first year in middle school in the movie *Diary of a Wimpy Kid*, based on a bestselling book series of the same name. At one point in his school year, Greg decides to audition for

the school musical, *The Wizard of Oz*. The music director, Mrs. Norton, chooses her favorite song for musical auditions: the 1983 pop hit "Total Eclipse of the Heart." Thus begins a montage of clips of the middle school students singing various parts of "Total Eclipse" completely out of tune while the camera occasionally focuses on Mrs. Norton, looking horrified . . . until Greg Heffley begins to sing the hook of the song, "And I need you more tonight / and I need you more than ever" perfectly in tune, loud, strong, and beautiful. Mrs. Norton looks absolutely thrilled.

MRS. NORTON

Greg Heffley! What a *lovely* soprano voice you have! I'm . . . I'm . . . *stunned! (a look of realization comes over her face) Maybe YOU should be Dorothy!*

Mrs. Norton goes on to say that his voice is too high for the other male roles, so she will cast him as a singing tree. Greg agrees, but only because he thinks that he will be able to throw apples at the girl playing Dorothy, his enemy, as the trees do in the film *The Wizard of Oz*.

- *The Music of Silence* (2017)
  This movie chronicles the life of professional singer Andrea Bocelli. During adolescence, young Andrea sings publicly during his voice change and is quite embarrassed. Although his family is supportive of him and recognizes that this is normal for a boy his age, he is incredibly frustrated because he feels that he let everyone down.
- *Harry Potter*
  Actor Rupert Grint made his first appearance as Ron Weasley in the *Harry Potter* movies in 2001 at the age of 11. The film series took place over the course of the next ten years, with the final film released in 2011. If you trace Ron across the films, you can hear that Grint's voice is changing as he progresses through adolescence, especially in the middle of the series.
  There were claims that Daniel Radcliff, who played Harry Potter, experienced voice change toward the end of filming *Harry Potter and the Sorcerer's Stone* (2001); he was 12 years old at that time. It was claimed that the filmmakers hired British actor Joe Sowerbutts to dub Radcliffe's voice in the final few scenes so there would be no voice cracking in the movie. (*Guardian*, November 1, 2001, https://www.theguardian.com/film/2001/nov/01/harrypotter.news)
  Representatives from Warner Brothers came forth and denied the story, saying that "the Hollywood studio said that 'no voice other than that of

Daniel Radcliffe' was used on the movie" (*Telegraph*, November 2, 2001, https://www.telegraph.co.uk/news/uknews/1361257/Studio-has-last-word-over-Harry-Potter-and-the-broken-voice.html). When you next watch this movie, keep a close ear out to see if you can determine the real story.

- Additional examples of voices that changed during production include:
  - o Bran Stark from *Game of Thrones*, actor Isaac Hempstead Wright
  - o Screech from *Saved by the Bell*, actor Dustin Diamond

CHAPTER 6

Additional resources regarding adolescent singers and their voices:

- Ashley, M. (2011). The angel enigma: Experienced boy singers' perceptual judgements of changing voices. *Music Education Research, 13*(3), 343–354.
- Ashley, M. (2013). The English choral tradition and the secular trend in boys' pubertal timing. *International Journal of Research in Choral Singing, 4*(2), 4–27.
- Bond, V. (2018). Like putting a circle with a square: A male alto's choral journey. In B. C. Talbot (Ed.), *Marginalized voices in music education* (pp. 137–152). New York: Routledge.
- Cooksey, J., Cox, N., & Hook, S. (1998). Changing voice and middle school music: An interview with John Cooksey and Nancy Cox. *Choral Journal, 39*(1), 21–26.
- Decoster, W., Ghesquiere, S., & Van Steenberg, S. (2008). Great talent, excellent voices—no problem for pubertal girls? *Logopedics, Phoniatrics, Vocology, 33*, 104–112.
- Elorriaga, A. (2018). *El sonido se transforma: Educación coral para adolescents.* [Sound transforms: Choral education for adolescents]. Editorial Anexo.
- Fisher, R. (2009). British and American theories of the changing male voice: An historical overview. *Journal of Historical Research in Music Education, 31*(1), 37–47.
- Fisher, R. A. (2010). Effect of ethnicity on the age of onset of the male voice change. *Journal of Research in Music Education, 58*(2), 116–130.
- Fisher, R. A. (2014). The impacts of the voice change, grade level, and experience on the singing self-efficacy of emerging adolescent males. *Journal of Research in Music Education, 62*(3), 277–290.

- Freer, P. K. (2009a). Choral warm-ups for changing adolescent voices. *Music Educators Journal, 95*(3), 57–62.
- Freer, P. K. (2009b). *Getting started with middle school choir* (2nd ed.). Lanham, MD: Rowman & Littlefield Education.
- Freer, P. K. (Ed.) (2012). The male choral singer: From adolescence to college. Part 1: From middle school to high school. [special themed issue.] *Choral Journal, 52* (9).
- Freer, P. K. (Ed.) (2012). The male choral singer: From adolescence to college. Part 2: From high school to college. [special themed issue.] *Choral Journal, 52* (10).
- Freer, P. K. (2012). From boys to men: Male choral singing in the United States. In S. Harrison & G. Welch (Eds.), *Perspectives on males and singing* (pp. 13–26). New York: Springer.
- Freer, P. K. (2015). Perspectives of European boys about their voice change and school choral singing: Developing the possible selves of adolescent male singers. *British Journal of Music Education, 32*(1), 87–106.
- Freer, P. K. (2016). The changing voices of male choristers: An enigma . . . to them. *Music Education Research, 18*(1), 74–90.
- Freer, P. K., & Elorriaga, A. (2017). El desarrollo de la voz masculina durante la adolescencia: Una pedagogía basada en la investigación [Toward a pedagogy informed by research about the boy's changing voice]. *Revista Española de Pedagogía, 75*(268), 463–480.
- Freer, P. K. (2018). Research-to-resources: Initial steps in vocal technique for boys experiencing difficulty with phonation during the adolescent voice change. *Update: Applications of Research in Music Education, 37*(1), 9–12.
- Killian, J. N., & Wayman, J. B. (2010). A descriptive study of vocal maturation among male adolescent vocalists and instrumentalists. *Journal of Research in Music Education, 58*(5), 5–19.
- Parker, E. (2014). The process of social identity development in adolescent high school choral singers: A grounded theory. *Journal of Research in Music Education, 62*(1), 18–32.
- Parker, E. (2018). A grounded theory of adolescent high school women's choir singers' process of social identity development. *Journal of Research in Music Education, 65*(4), 439–460.
- Phillips, K. H. (2014). *Teaching kids to sing* (2nd ed.). Boston Schirmer.
- Phillips, K. H. (2016). *Directing the choral music program* (2nd ed.). New York: Oxford University Press.
- Professor Martin Ashley's website, for access to his research: www.martin-ashley.com

- Shaw, J. (2012). The skin that we sing: Culturally responsive choral music education. *Music Educators Journal, 98*(4), 75–81.
- Shaw, J. (2016). "The music I was meant to sing": Adolescent choral students' perceptions of culturally responsive pedagogy. *Journal of Research in Music Education, 64*(1), 45–70.
- Stockton, P. (2015). Irvin Cooper (1900–1971) and the development of the cambiata concept for adolescent changing voices. *Journal of Historical Research in Music Education, 37*(1), 75–87.
- Swanson, F. J. (1960). When voices change: An experiment in junior high school music. *Music Educators Journal, 46*(4), 50–56.
- Swanson, F. J. (1961). The proper care and feeding of changing voices. *Music Educators Journal,* 48(2), 63–66.
- Sweet, B. (2016, April). *Choral Journal* and the adolescent female changing voice. *Choral Journal, 56*(9), 53–64.
- Sweet, B. (2016, October). Keeping the glass half full: Teaching adolescents with a holistic perspective. *Choral Journal, 57*(3), 6–14.
- Thurman, L. (1988). Vocal health and choral singing: When voice classifications limit singing ability. *Choral Journal, 28*(10), 25–33.
- van Gend, M., Matthias, P., Scott, N., & Allan, C. (2017). Adolescent girls' changing voices: Re-thinking classification. *Australian Voice, 18,* 1–13.

Additional resources to support LGBTQ+ students in music:

- A Guide for Supporting Transgender Students in K-12 Schools: https://www.genderspectrum.org/staging/wp-content/uploads/2015/08/Schools-in-Transition-2015.pdf
- Aguirre, R. (2018). Finding the trans voice: A review of the literature on accommodating transgender singers. *Update: Applications of Research in Music Education, 37*(1), 36–41.
- Ahad-Legardy, B., & Poon, O. A. (2018). *Difficult subjects: Insights and strategies for teaching about race, sexuality, and gender.* Sterling, VA: Stylus.
- Bartolome, S. J., & Stanford, M. E. (2018). "Can't I sing with the girls?" A transgender music educator's journey. In B. C. Talbot (Ed.), *Marginalized voices in music education* (pp. 114–136). New York: Routledge.
- Bergonzi, L. (2009). Sexual orientation and music education: Continuing a tradition. *Music Educators Journal, 96*(2), 21–25.
- Garrett, M. L. (2012). The LGBTQ component of 21st-century music teacher training: Strategies for inclusion from the research literature. *Update: Applications of Research in Music Education, 31*(1), 55–62.
- Jackson Hearns, L., & Kremer, B. (2018). *The singing teacher's guide to transgender voices*. San Diego, CA: Plural Publishing.

- Kosciw, J. G., Greytak, E. A., Bartklewicz, M. J., Boesen, M. J., & Palmer, N. A. (2012). *The 2011 National School Climate Survey: The experiences of lesbian, gay, bisexual and transgender youth in our nation's schools.* New York: Gay, Lesbian & Straight Education Network.
- Manternach, B. (2017). Teaching transgender singers. Part 2: The singers' perspectives. *Journal of Singing, 74*(2), 209–214.
- Manternach, B., Chipman, M., Rainero, R., & Stave, C. (2017). Teaching transgender singers. Part 1: The voice teachers' perspectives. *Journal of Singing, 74*(1), 83–88.
- Musicians to explore: Namoli Brennet, Mya Byrne, Mina Caputo, Ryan Cassata, Eli Conley, Beth Elliott, Marie France, Laura Jane Grace, Romy Haag, Antony Hegarty, Christine Jorgensen, Katastrophe, Skylar Kergil, Amanda Lepore, Bell Nuntita, Richard O'Brien, Kim Petras, Ruth Pearce, Nomi Ruiz, Lucas Silveira, Breanna Sinclairé, T. Thomason, and Ramon Te Wake
- Nichols, J. (2013). Rie's story, Ryan's journey: Music in the life of a transgender student. *Journal of Research in Music Education, 61*(3), 262–279.
- Palkki, J. (2015). Gender trouble: Males, adolescence, and masculinity in the choral context. *Choral Journal, 56*(4), 24–35.
- Palkki, J. (2016). *"My voice speaks for itself": The experiences of three transgender students in secondary school choral programs.* Doctoral dissertation, Michigan State University, East Lansing.
- Palkki, J. (2017). Inclusivity in action: Transgender students in the choral classroom. *Choral Journal, 57*(11), 20–34.
- Palkki, J., & Caldwell, P. (2017). "We are often invisible": A survey on safe space for LGBTQ students in secondary school choral programs. *Research Studies in Music Education, 40*(1), 28–49.
- Sieck, S. (2017). *Teaching with respect: Inclusive pedagogy for choral directors.* Milwaukee, WI: Hal Leonard.
- Silveira, J. M. (2019). Perspectives of a transgender music education student. *Journal of Research in Music Education, 66*(4), 428–448.
- Silveira, J. M., & Goff, S. C. (2016). Music teachers' attitudes towards transgender students and supportive school practices. *Journal of Research in Music Education, 64*(2), 138–158.
- Transgender Unicorn: http://www.transstudent.org/gender

REFERENCES

Abitbol, J., & Abitbol, P. (2014). The larynx: A hormonal target. In J. S. Rubin, R. T. Sataloff, & G. S. Korovin (Eds.), *Diagnosis and treatment of voice disorders* (4th ed., pp. 431–455). San Diego, CA: Plural Publishing.

Abitbol, J., Abitbol, P., & Abitbol, B. (1999). Sex hormones and the female voice. *Journal of Voice, 13*(3), 424–446.

Abitbol, J., de Brux, J., Millot, G., Masson, M-F., Mimoun, O. L., Pau, H., & Abitbol, B. (1989). Does a hormonal vocal cord cycle exist in women? Study of vocal premenstrual syndrome in voice performers by videostroboscopy-glottography and cytology on 38 women. *Journal of Voice, 3*(2), 157–162.

Alison, R., & Clifford, J. (Producers), & King, P. (Director). 2018. *Paddington 2* [Motion picture]. Burbank, CA: Warner Bros. Pictures.

Asher, J. J., & Garcia, R. (1969). The optimal age to learn a foreign language. *The Modern Language Journal, 53*(5), 334–341.

Banks, E., & Brooks, P. (Producers), & Moore, J. (Director). (2012). *Pitch perfect* [Motion picture]. : Universal Pictures.

Barlow, C. A., & Howard, D. M. (2002). Voice source changes of child and adolescent subjects undergoing singing training: A preliminary study. *Logopedics, Phoniatrics, Vocology, 27*, 66–73.

Baudrillard, J. (1994). *Simulacra and simulation*. Ann Arbor: University of Michigan Press.

Behnke, E., & Browne, L. (1885). *The child's voice*. Chicago: A. N. Marquis.

Bishop, G. J. (2017). *Unfu*k yourself: Get out of your head and into your life*. New York: HarperCollins.

Bowers, J. (2008). Building early choral experiences: Part Two—The middle school choral program. In M. Holt & J. Jordan (Eds.), *The school choral program: Philosophy, planning, organizing, and teaching* (pp. 359–374). Chicago: GIA Publications.

Brown, B. (2012). *Daring greatly: How the courage to be vulnerable transforms the way we live, love, parent, and lead*. New York: Penguin Group.

Brown, K. M. (2015). Sex hormones and the female voice: Communication in the voice studio. *Journal of Singing, 71*(4), 447–456.

Chapman, J. L. (2012). *Singing and teaching singing: A holistic approach to classical voice*. San Diego: Plural Publishing.

Clements, R., & Musker, J. (Directors). (1989). *The little mermaid* [Motion picture]. : Walt Disney Pictures/Silver Screen Partners IV.

Collins, D. L. (1999). *Teaching choral music* (2nd ed.). Upper Saddle River, NJ: Prentice Hall.

Cooksey, J. M. (1977a). The development of a contemporary, eclectic theory for the training and cultivation of the junior high school male changing voice: Part 1, Existing theories. *Choral Journal, 18*(2), 5–14.
Cooksey, J. M. (1977b). The development of a contemporary, eclectic theory for the training and cultivation of the junior high school male changing voice: Part 2, Scientific and empirical findings; Some tentative solutions. *Choral Journal, 18*(3), 5–16.
Cooksey, J. M. (1977c). The development of a contemporary, eclectic theory for the training and cultivation of the junior high school male changing voice: Part 3, Developing an integrated approach to the care and training of the junior high school male changing voice. *Choral Journal, 18*(4), 5–15.
Cooksey, J. M. (1978). The development of a contemporary, eclectic theory for the training and cultivation of the junior high school male changing voice: Part 4, Selecting music for the junior high school male changing voice. *Choral Journal, 18*(5), 5–17.
Cooksey, J. M. (1992). *Working with the adolescent voice.* St. Louis, MO: Concordia Publishing House.
Cooksey, J. M. (1999). *Working with adolescent voices.* St. Louis, MO: Concordia Publishing House.
Cooper, I., & Kuersteiner, K. O (1965). *Teaching junior high school music.* Boston: Allyn and Bacon.
Coverdale, D., & Marsden, B. (1982). Here I go again [Recorded by Whitesnake]. On *Saints & Sinners*. Burbank, CA: Geffen/Warner Bros.
Daw, S. F. (1970). Age of boys' puberty in Leipzig, 1727-49, as indicated by voice breaking in J. S. Bach's choir members. *Human Biology, 42*(1), 87–89.
Deak, J., & Deak, T. (2013). *The owner's manual for driving your adolescent brain.* San Francisco: Little Pickle Press.
Del Vecho, P. (Producer), & Lee, J., & Buck, C. (Directors). 2013. *Frozen* [Motion picture]. Burbank, CA: Walt Disney Animation Studios.
Dickens, C. (1843). *A Christmas carol in prose, being a ghost-story of Christmas.* London: Chapman & Hall.
Docter, P. (Director), & Lasseter, J., & Stanton, A. (Producers). (2015). *Inside out* [Motion picture]. Emeryville, CA: Pixar Animation Studios.
Duckworth, A. (2016). *Grit: The power of passion and perseverance.* New York: Scribner.
Eby, T. L., & Nadol, J. B. (1986). Postnatal growth of the human temporal bone: Implications for cochlear implants in children. *Annals of Otology, Rhinology, and Laryngology, 95*(4), 356–364.
Elorriaga, A. (2011). The construction of male gender identity through choir singing at a Spanish secondary school. *International Journal of Music Education, 29*, 318–332. doi: 10.1177/0255761411421091.
Fabienne. (2016, Jan 12). *Ethereal voices from Tirol: The Wilten Boys' Choir* [Web blog post]. Retrieved from https://www.blog.tirol/en/2016/12/ethereal-voices-from-tirol-the-wilten-boys-choir/
Finn, W. J. (1939). *The art of the choral conductor.* Boston: C. C. Birchard.
Freer, P. K. (2006). Hearing the voices of adolescent boys in choral music: A self-story. *Research Studies in Music Education, 27*, 69–81. doi: 10.1177/1321103X060270010501.
Freer, P. K. (2009). "I'll sing with my buddies": Fostering the possible selves of male choral singers. *International Journal of Music Education, 27*, 341–355. doi: 10.1177/0255761409345918.

Freer, P. K. (2010). Foundation of the boy's expanding voice: A response to Henry Leck. *Choral Journal, 50*(7), 29–35.

Gackle, L. (1991). The adolescent female voice: Characteristics of change and stages of development. *Choral Journal, 31*(8), 17–25.

Gackle, L. (2006). Finding Ophelia's voice: The female voice during adolescence. *Choral Journal, 47*(5), 28–37.

Gackle, L. (2011). *Finding Ophelia's voice, opening Ophelia's heart*. Dayton, OH: Heritage Music Press.

Gates, R., Forrest, L. A., & Obert, K. (2013). *The owner's manual to the voice: A guide for singers and other professional voice users*. New York: Oxford University Press.

Goldberg, A., & Firek, M. (Writers), & Katzenberg, D. (Director). (2015, Sept 30). A chorus lie [Television series episode]. In A. Barnow (Producer), *The Goldbergs*. Culver City, CA: Sony Picture Studios.

Grant, A. J., Reynolds, D., Sermon, W., McKee, B., & Platzman, D. (2012). On top of the world [Recorded by Imagine Dragons.] On *Night Visions*. Santa Monica, CA: Interscope Records.

Grohl, D., Hawkins, T., Mendel, N., & Shiflett, C. (2003). Times like these [Recorded by Foo Fighters]. On *One by One*. New York: RCA.

Hall, A., Cobb, R., Kapoor, K., Kuchai, R., & Sandhu, G. (2017). The instrument of voice: The "true" vocal cord or vocal fold? *Journal of Voice, 31*(2), 133–134.

Harris, R. L. (1987). The young female voice and alto. *Choral Journal, 28*(3), 21–22.

Heman-Ackah, Y. D., Sataloff, R. T., & Hawkshaw, M. J. (2013). *A medical guide for achieving and maintaining a healthy voice*. Narberth, PA: Science & Medicine.

Hirano, M. (1981). *Clinical examination of voice*. New York: Springer-Verlag.

Jensen, F. E. (2015). *The teenage brain: A neuroscientist's survival guide to raising adolescents and young adults*. New York: HarperCollins.

Jordan, L. (Director). (1999). *Eddie Izzard: Dressed to kill* [Televised comedy special]. Tel Aviv–Yafo, Israel: Ella Communications Ltd.

Kadakia, S., Carlson, D., & Sataloff, R. T. (2013). The effect of hormones on the voice. *Journal of Singing, 69*(5), 571–574.

Kahane, J. C. (1982). Growth of the human prepubertal and pubertal larynx. *Journal of Speech and Hearing Research, 25*, 446–455.

Keefe, D. H., Bulen, J. C., Arehart, K. H., & Burns, E. M. (1993). Ear-canal impedance and reflection coefficient in human infants and adults. *Journal of the Acoustical Society of America, 94*(5), 2617–2638.

Kennedy, M. A. (2002). "It's cool because we like to sing": Junior high school boys' experience of choral music as an elective. *Research Studies in Music Education, 18*, 26–36. doi: 10.1177/1321103X020180010401.

Kennedy, M. C. (2004). "It's a metaphorphosis": Guiding the voice change at the American Boychoir School. *Journal of Research in Music Education, 52*, 264–280. doi: 10.2307/3345859.

Killian, J. (1997). Perceptions of the voice-change process: Male adult versus adolescent musicians and nonmusicians. *Journal of Research in Music Education, 45*, 521–535. doi: 10.2307/3345420.

Kinberg, S. (Producer), & Leitch, D. (Director). 2018. *Deadpool 2* [Motion picture]. USA: Twentieth Century Fox.

Kinney, J. (2007). *Diary of a wimpy kid*. New York: Amulet Books.

Klinefelter syndrome. (n.d.). *Klinefelter syndrome information and support*. Retrieved from http://www.klinefeltersyndrome.org/

Krizman, J., Tierney, A., Fitzroy, A. B., Skoe, E., Amar, J., & Kraus, N. (2015). Continued maturation of auditory brainstem function during adolescence: A longitudinal approach. *Clinical Neurophysiology, 126*, 2348–2355.

Kruse, A. (2016). Featherless dinosaurs and the hip-hop simulacrum: Reconsidering hip-hop's appropriateness for the music classroom. *Music Educators Journal, 102*(4), 13–21.

Lesko, N. (2012). *Act your age! A cultural construction of adolescence*. New York: Taylor & Francis.

Litovsky, R. (2015). Development of the auditory system. *Handbook of Clinical Neurology, 129*, 55–72.

Luchsinger, R., & Arnold, G. E. (1965). *Voice-speech-language: Clinical communicology; Its physiology and pathology*. Belmont, CA: Wadsworth.

Mariall, C., & Rossman, G. B. (2011). *Designing qualitative research* (5th ed.). Thousand Oaks, CA: Sage.

Marlens, N., & Black, C. (Writers), & McBride, J. (Director). (1990, Feb 27). The glee club [Television series episode]. In B. Brush (Producer), *The wonder years*. Burbank, CA: New World Television, The Black/Marlens Company.

Mathieson, L. (2001). *The voice & its disorders* (6th ed.). London: Whurr Publishers Ltd.

McKenzie, D. (1956). *Training the boy's changing voice*. New Brunswick, NJ: Rutgers University Press.

McKim, D. (Producer), & Anderson, S. J. (Director). (2007). *Meet the Robinsons* [Motion picture]. Burbank, CA: Walt Disney Pictures.

McMahan, I. (2008). *Adolescence*. Boston, MA: Pearson.

Minax, M. (Director). (2010). *Riot acts* [Motion picture on Amazon Video]. Outcast Films.

Mitchell, M., & Dohrn, W. (Directors). (2016). *Trolls* [Motion picture]. 20th Century Fox.

Moller, H. (1985). Voice change in human biological development. *Journal of Interdisciplinary History, 16*(2), 239–253.

Northern, J. L., & Downs, M. P. (1984). *Hearing in children*. Baltimore: Williams & Wilkins.

Oberlander, E. (2010). Premenstrual syndrome and its effect on laryngeal functionality: An approach for singers and pedagogues. *Journal of Singing, 67*(1), 27–34.

Obituary: Emil Behnke. (1892, Oct 1). *Musical Times and Singing Class Circular, 33*(596), 605. Retrieved from http://www.jstor.org/stable/3362429

Obituary: Lennox Browne. (1902, Dec). *Journal of Laryngology, Rhinology, and Otology, 17*(12), 629–631. Retrieved from https://www.cambridge.org/core/services/aop-cambridge-core/content/view/E8F7F770EEFD25DB9FADF6BB9FB4F50E/S1755146300172105a.pdf/lennox-browne-f-r-c-s-e.pdf

Obituary: John Marion Cooksey. (2012, Nov 3). *Deseret News*. Retrieved from http://www.legacy.com/obituaries/deseretnews/obituary.aspx?n=john-marion-cooksey&pid=160786996

O'Toole, P. (1994). "I sing in a choir, but I have 'no voice!'" *Quarterly Journal of Music Teaching and Learning, 4–5*(5–1), 65–77.

O'Toole, P. (2000). Why I don't feel included in these musics or matters. *Bulletin of the Council for Research in Music Education, 144*, 28–39.

O'Toole, P. (2005). "I sing in a choir, but I have 'no voice!'" *Visions of Research in Music Education, 6*, 1–26. http://www-usr.rider.edu/~vrme/

Pacific Boychoir Academy. (2018). "Branded name vocal training." Retrieved from http://www.pacificboychoir.org/day-school/troubadors

Parker, E. C. (2014). The process of social identity development in adolescent high school choral singers: A grounded theory. *Journal of Research in Music Education, 62*, 18–32. doi: 10.1177/0022429413520009.

Patton, M. Q. (2015). *Qualitative research & evaluation methods* (4th ed.). Thousand Oaks, CA: Sage.

Plotkin, H., & Jackson, K. R. (Producers), & Lasseter, J. (Director). (1999). *Toy Story 2* [Motion picture]. Emeryville, CA: Pixar Animation Studios.

Rosen, M. (1989). *We're going on a bear hunt.* New York: Margaret K. McElderry Books.

Rundus, K. (2009). *Cantabile: A manual about beautiful singing for singers, teachers of singing and choral Conductors.* San Pedro, CA: Pavane Publishing.

Sataloff, R. T., Emerich, K. A., & Hoover, C. A. (1997). Endocrine dysfunction. In R. R. Sataloff (Ed.), *Professional voice: The science and art of clinical care* (2nd ed., pp. 291–297). San Diego: Singular Publishing Group.

Schrobsdorff, S. (2016, Nov 7). The kids are not all right. *Time, 188*(19), 44–51.

Schwartz, S., & Starr, B. (Writers), & Baron, A. (Director). (1972, Jan14). Dough, re, mi [Television series episode]. In H. Leed (Producer), *The Brady Bunch.* Los Angeles: Paramount Studios.

Sex chromosome. (n.d.). In *Encyclopaedia Brittanica's online encyclopedia.* Retrieved from https://www.britannica.com/science/sex-chromosome

Shore, D. (2004–2012). *House* [Television series]. Los Angeles: Fox Broadcasting Company.

Siegel, D. J. (2015). *Brainstorm: The power and purpose of the teenage brain.* New York: Jeremy P. Tarcher/Penguin.

Skoe, E., & Kraus, N. (2013). Musical training heightens auditory brainstem function during sensitive periods in development. *Frontiers in Psychology, 4,* 622.

Standring, S. (Ed.). (2016). *Gray's anatomy: The anatomical basis of clinical practice* (41st ed.). New York: Elsevier Limited.

Steinberg, L. (2014). *Age of opportunity: Lessons from the new science of adolescence.* New York: Houghton Mifflin Harcourt.

Stiles, H. D. W. (2017). Voice trainer, Emile Behnke, "as accurate as Huxley and as fascinating as Faraday." *UCL Ear Institute & Action on Hearing Loss Libraries.* Retrieved from http://blogs.ucl.ac.uk/library-rnid/2017/02/17/voice-trainer-emil-behnke-as-accurate-as-huxley-and-as-fascinating-as-faraday/

Sussman, E. S. (2013). Attention matters: Pitch vs. pattern processing in adolescence. *Frontiers in Psychology, 4*(333), 1–8.

Swanson, F. J. (1973). *Music teaching in the junior high and middle school.* New York: Meredith Corporation.

Swanson, F. J. (1977). *The male singing voice ages eight to eighteen.* Cedar Rapids, IA: Laurance Press.

Swanson, F. J. (1984). Changing voices: Don't leave out the boys. *Music Educators Journal, 70*(5), 47–50.

Sweet, B. (2014). Qualitative choral music research. In C. Conways (Ed.), *The Oxford Handbook of Qualitative Research in American Music Education* (pp. 429–447). New York: Oxford University Press.

Sweet, B. (2015). The adolescent female changing voice: A phenomenological investigation. *Journal of Research in Music Education, 63*(1), 70–88.

Sweet, B. (2016a). *Growing musicians: Teaching music in middle school and beyond.* New York: Oxford University Press.

Sweet. B. (2016b, Feb 9). Adolescents and adolescence: The glass really is half-full. [Web log comment]. Retrieved from https://blog.oup.com/2016/02/adolescent-music-education-compassion/

Sweet, B. (2018). Voice change and singing experiences of adolescent females. *Journal of Research in Music Education, 66*(2), 133–149.

Sweet, B., & Bergonzi, L. (2016a, May 19). Adolescent voice change: Enriching the conversation with transgender perspectives. 3rd Symposium on LGBT Studies and Music Education, University of Illinois at Urbana-Champaign, Urbana.

Sweet, B., & Bergonzi, L. (2016b, July 28). Adolescent voice change: Enriching the conversation with transgender perspectives. 32nd World Conference of the International Society for Music Education, Glasgow, Scotland.

Sweet, B., Martin, E., & Bergonzi, L. (2016, Jan 29). Adolescent voice change: Enriching the conversation with transgender perspectives. Illinois Music Education Association All-State Conference, Peoria.

Sweet, B., & Parker, E. C. (2018). Female vocal identity: A phenomenology. *Journal of Research in Music Education, 67*(1), 62–82.

Tierney, A. T., Krizman, J., & Kraus, N. (2015). Music training alters the course of adolescent auditory development. *Proceedings of the National Academy of Sciences of the United States of America, 112*(32), 10062–10067.

Tierney, A., Krizman, J., Skoe, E., Johnston, K., & Krause, N. (2013). High school music classes enhance the neural processing of speech. *Frontiers in Psychology, 4*(855), 1–7.

Trevorrow, C. (Director). (2015). *Jurassic world* [Motion picture]. : Universal Pictures/ Amblin Entertainment.

Turner syndrome. (n.d.). *Turner syndrome society of the United States*. Retrieved from http://www.turnersyndrome.org/

Unkrich, L. (Director), & Lasseter, J. (Producer). (2017). *Coco*. Emeryville, CA: Pixar Animation Studios.

Verbinski, G. (Director). (2003). *Pirates of the Caribbean: The curse of the Black Pearl* [Motion picture]. USA: Walt Disney Pictures & Jerry Bruckheimer Films.

Vigil, P. (2015). Hormones and the female voice: An exploration of the female hormonal cycle from puberty to menopause and how it affects the vocal apparatus (Doctoral dissertation). Temple University, Philadelphia.

Watanabe, D., Savion-Lemieux, T., & Penhune, V. B. (2007). The effect of early musical training on adult motor performance: Evidence for a sensitive period in motor learning. *Experimental Brain Research, 176*(2), 332–340.

Weiss, D. (1950). The pubertal change of the human voice. *Folia Phoniatrica, 2*(3), 126–159.

Yanagisawa, E., Yanagisawa, K., & Sims, H. S. (2014). Videography and photography of the larynx. In J. S. Rubin, R. T. Sataloff, & G. S. Korovin (Eds.), *Diagnosis and treatment of voice disorders* (4th ed., pp. 303–319). San Diego: Plural Publishing.

INDEX

For the benefit of digital users, indexed terms that span two pages (e.g., 52–53) may, on occasion, appear on only one of those pages.

Note: Figures are indicated by *f* following the page number

The manufacturer's authorised representative in the EU for product safety is Oxford University Press España S.A. of El Parque Empresarial San Fernando de Henares, Avenida de Castilla, 2 – 28830 Madrid (www.oup.es/en or product.safety@oup.com). OUP España S.A. also acts as importer into Spain of products made by the manufacturer.

Printed in the USA/Agawam, MA
May 22, 2025

887900.056